# The Hibiscus Retreat:
# A Companion for Home, Wellness and Joy

**The Hibiscus Retreat:
A Companion for Home, Wellness and Joy**

ISBN 978-1-989647-30-1

© 2023 Olivia Taylor and Samantha Porter
A Byrd Press Publication
Toronto
www.byrdpress.com
publisher@byrdpress.com

Art Direction Felipe Silva

Dedicated to Charles Edward Telfair (1778-1833)

Charles Edward Telfair (1778-1833) was an Irish botanist known for his significant contributions to the field of botany. He was born in Belfast and later moved to Mauritius, where he made a lasting impact on the island's flora and botanical knowledge. Telfair was involved in cross-pollinating native species with forms of Hibiscus rosa-sinensis, which is considered "the most important genetic parent" of hibiscus. His work with hibiscus and other plant species has left a lasting legacy, and he is commemorated by the plant genus Telfairia, the lizard species Leiolopisma telfairii (Telfair's skink), and the mammal species Echinops telfairi (lesser hedgehog tenrec). Telfair's contributions to botany and his efforts to improve the education and housing of estate slaves in Mauritius have solidified his place in botanical history. His wife, Annabella Chamberlain, was also a botanical artist and plant collector, and some of her illustrations appeared in Curtis Botanical Magazine between 1826 and 1830. Telfair's collections were donated to the Zoological Society of London, but were dispersed and effectively lost when sold in 1855. His legacy continues to be celebrated, and the Charles Telfair Institute in Mauritius was renamed in his honor

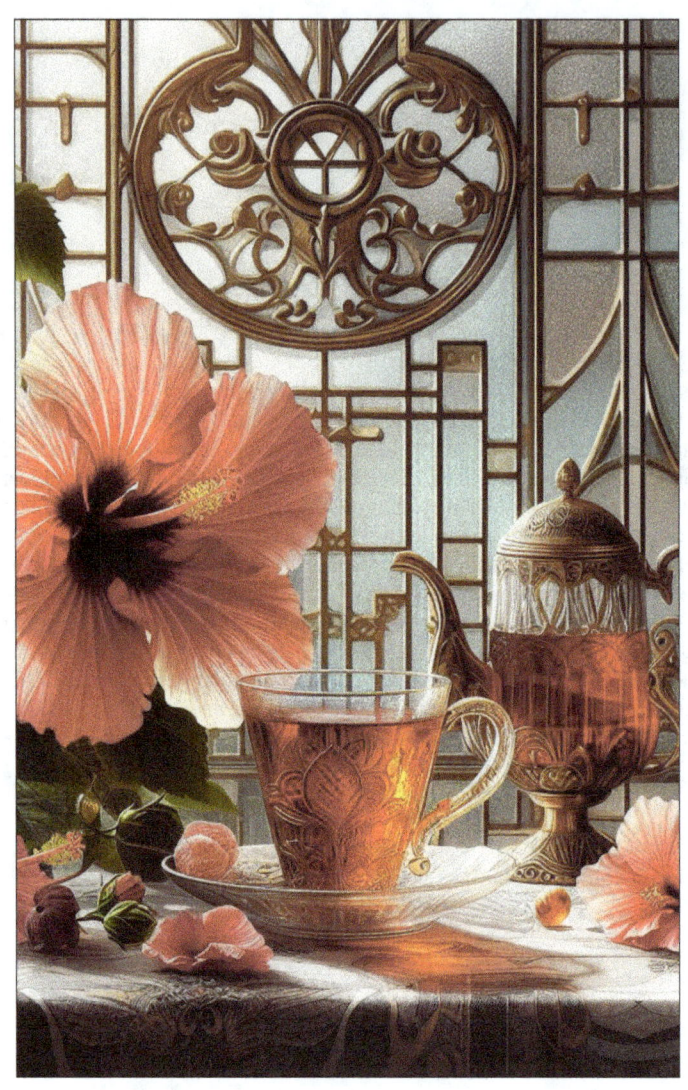

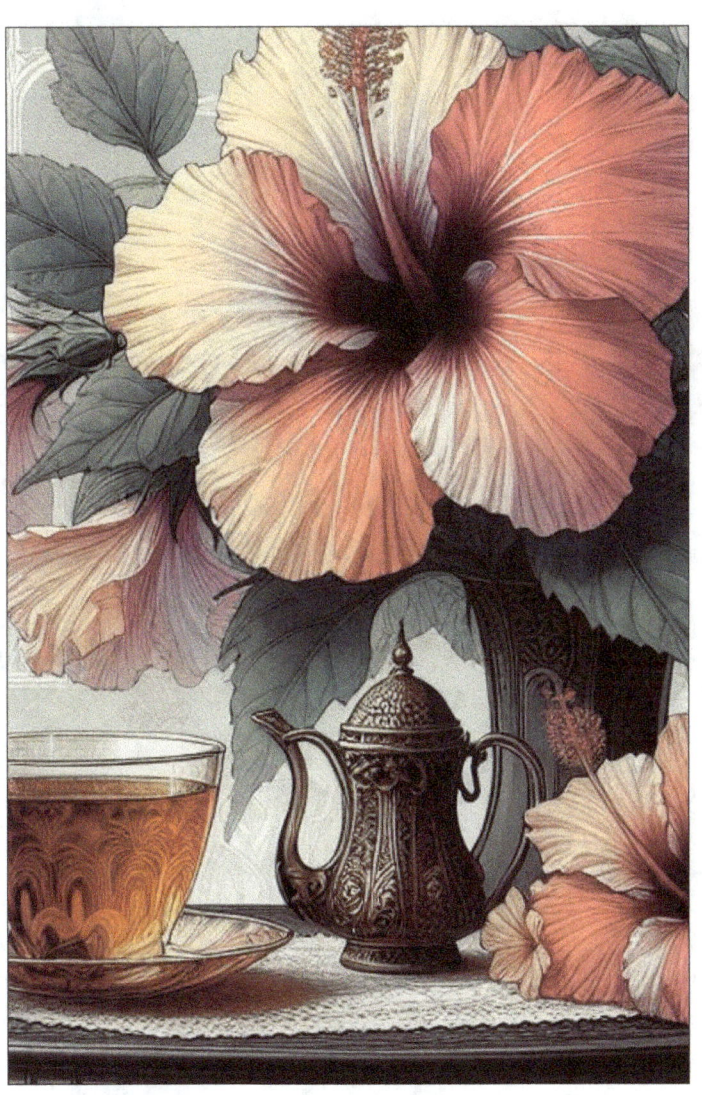

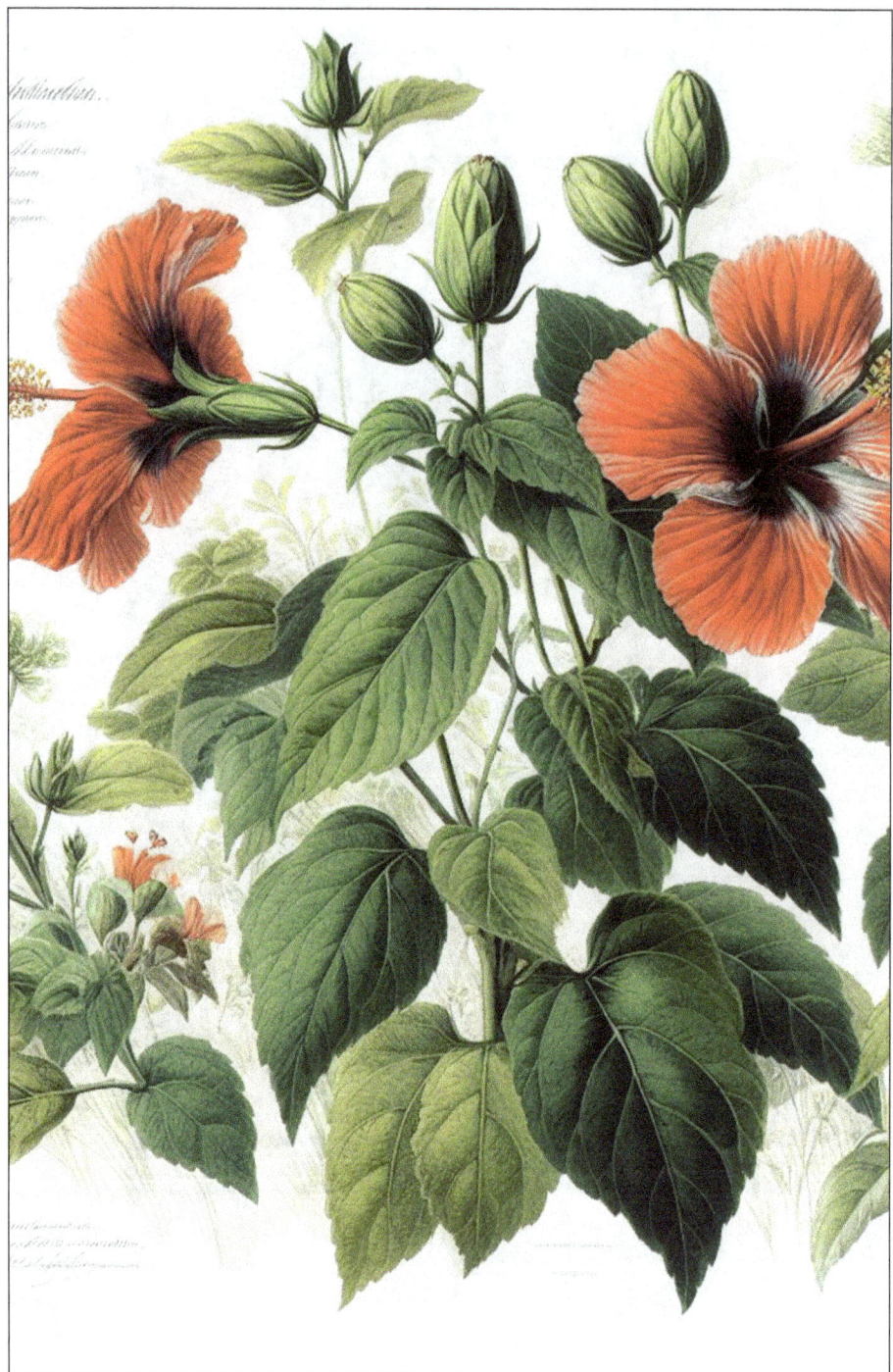

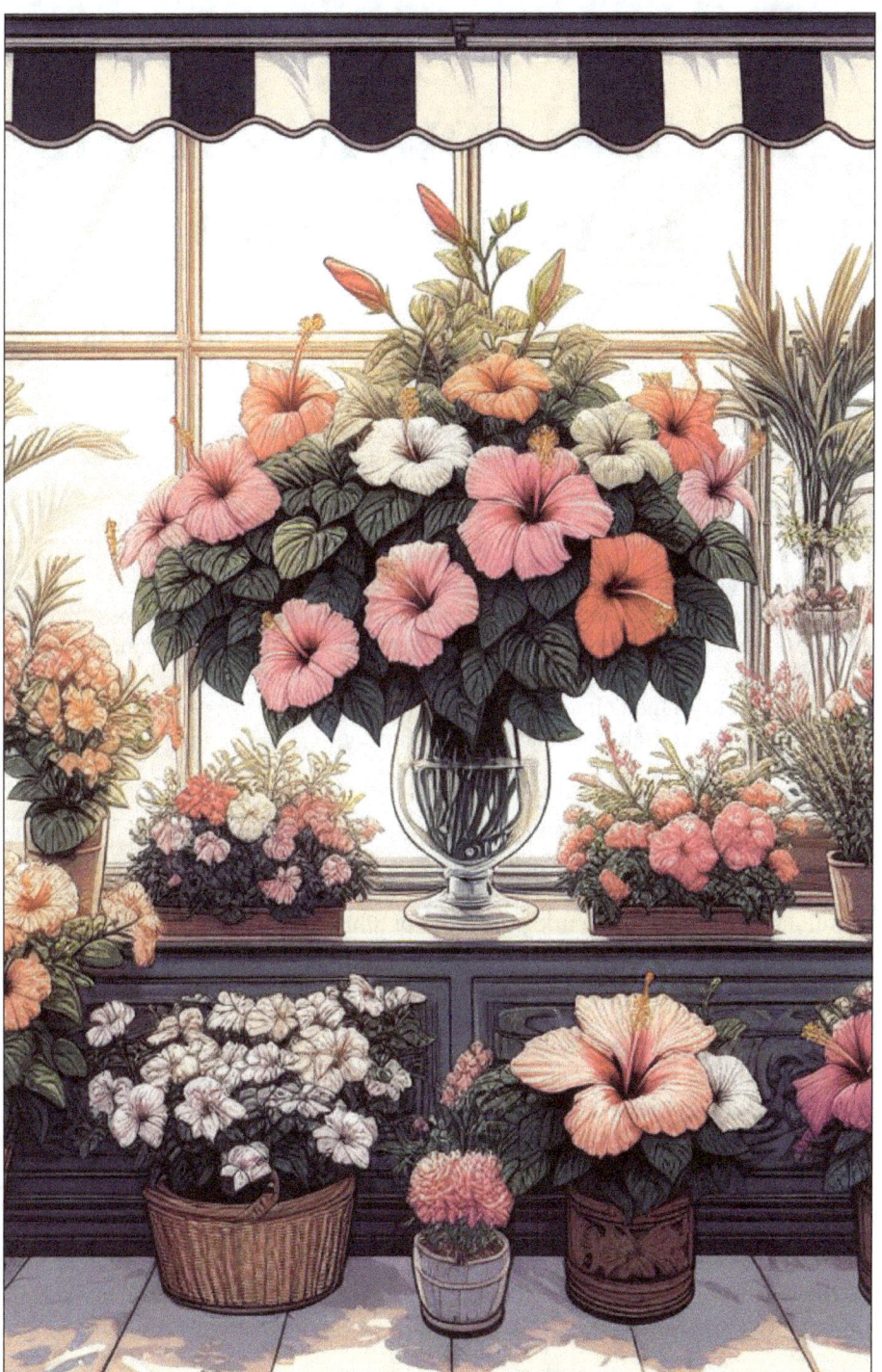

# Embracing Hibiscus: A Global Journey from Petal to Palate

From the sun-kissed landscapes of tropical havens to the arid regions of Africa, the story of hibiscus unfolds as a global odyssey intertwined with history, culture, and the intricate dance of trade routes. As we delve into the question of "Why Hibiscus?" we unveil a narrative that traverses continents, spans centuries, and underscores the botanical marvel that has become a cherished companion in our lives.

Historical Reverence:
The roots of hibiscus in human history run deep, dating back to ancient civilizations that recognized its beauty and therapeutic properties. Across cultures, hibiscus has been a symbol of love, prosperity, and celebration. In Ancient Egypt, it was associated with divine beauty, while in China, it found a place in traditional medicine. The vibrant petals have adorned ceremonies and rituals, echoing the rich tapestry of human heritage.

Culinary and Medicinal Tapestry:
As we fast forward to the present, hibiscus has seamlessly integrated itself into the culinary world, gracing tables from Cairo to California. Its infusion, be it in teas, beverages, or culinary creations, brings a burst of color and a delightful tartness. Simultaneously, the therapeutic properties of hibiscus, rich in antioxidants and vitamin C, have positioned it as a natural ally in promoting health and well-being.

A Global Harvest:
The journey of hibiscus products begins in lush plantations where these vibrant flowers bloom. From the fields of Sudan to the hillsides of Jamaica, the cultivation of hibiscus is an art passed down through generations. The meticulous harvesting of petals heralds the start of a logistical journey that spans continents. In regions like West Africa, where hibiscus cultivation is a livelihood, the industry becomes a vital economic force, connecting farmers to global markets.

The Logistics Unveiled:
As the petals are carefully plucked, they embark on a journey that involves drying, processing, and packaging. In the heart of hibiscus production, the

industry becomes a complex network of farmers, processors, and exporters. Logistics companies weave a tapestry that navigates regulatory landscapes, quality standards, and international trade dynamics. From the fields to your home, hibiscus undergoes a meticulous journey that ensures the freshness and quality retained in every petal.

Sustainable Practices:
The hibiscus industry is also evolving with a keen eye on sustainability. Many regions are embracing eco-friendly cultivation practices, ensuring that the global demand for hibiscus does not compromise the delicate ecosystems that nurture these blossoms. Sustainable farming practices, fair trade initiatives, and community empowerment are becoming integral aspects of the hibiscus journey, making it not just a commodity but a catalyst for positive change.

Culinary and Cultural Fusion:
In the kitchens of renowned chefs and the homes of enthusiasts, hibiscus becomes a versatile muse. Its floral notes inspire mixologists to craft inventive cocktails, and its rich color elevates culinary creations. The fusion of hibiscus into global cuisines is a testament to its adaptability, inviting people worldwide to savor its unique charm.

In essence, the allure of hibiscus is a convergence of nature's beauty, historical reverence, and the intricate interplay of global trade. Its journey from fields to tables is a story of resilience, adaptation, and a shared appreciation for the diversity it brings to our lives. So, why hibiscus? Because in its petals, we find not just a flower but a global ambassador, weaving together histories, cultures, and the joy of discovery.

Within, we seek to provide an accessible fun introduction to working with and enjoying one of the most iconic and cherish flowers in the world. Enjoy!

# Table of Contents

| | | |
|---|---|---|
| I. | Drinks | 1 |
| II. | Smoothies | 16 |
| III. | Mocktails & Cocktails | 34 |
| IV. | Tinctures and Elixirs | 56 |
| V. | Hibiscus Home Spa | 72 |
| VI. | Hibiscus Household | 100 |
| VII. | Hibiscus Gifts And Celebrations | 110 |
| VIII. | Final Thoughts | 120 |
| IX. | Index of Recipes, Formulas and Procedures | 124 |

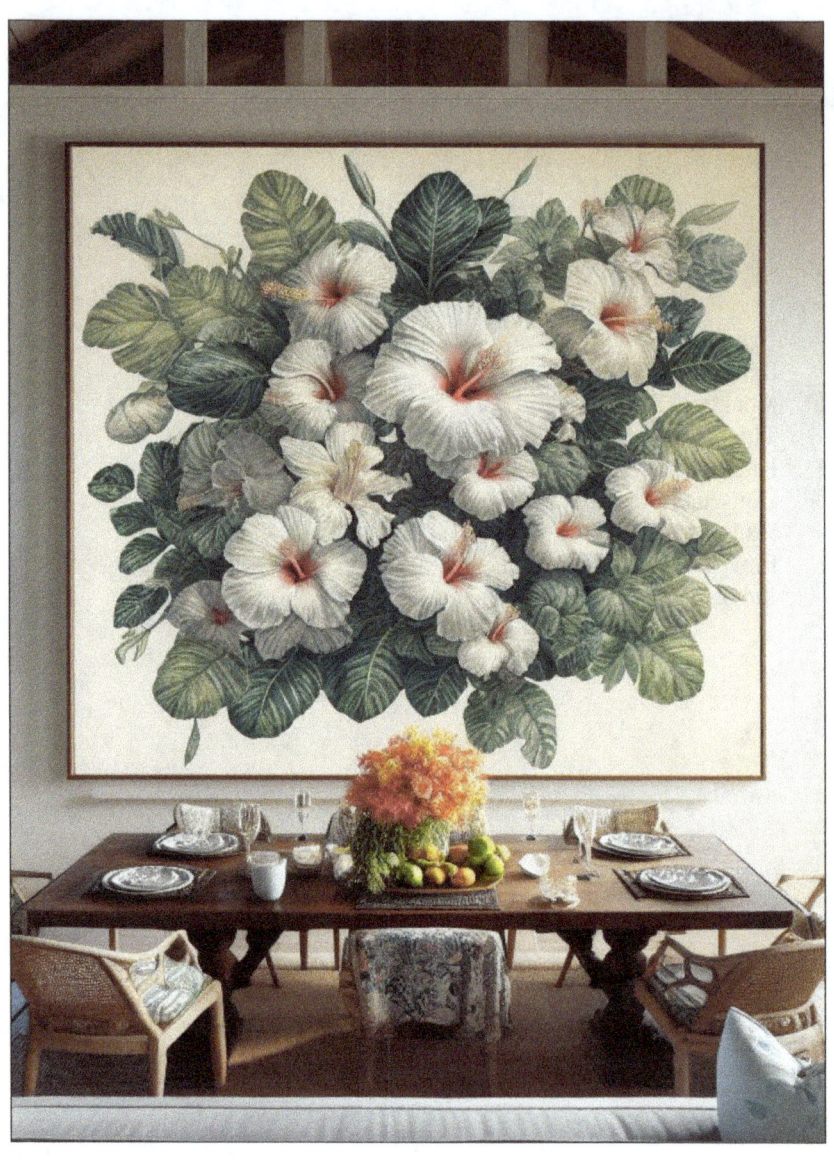

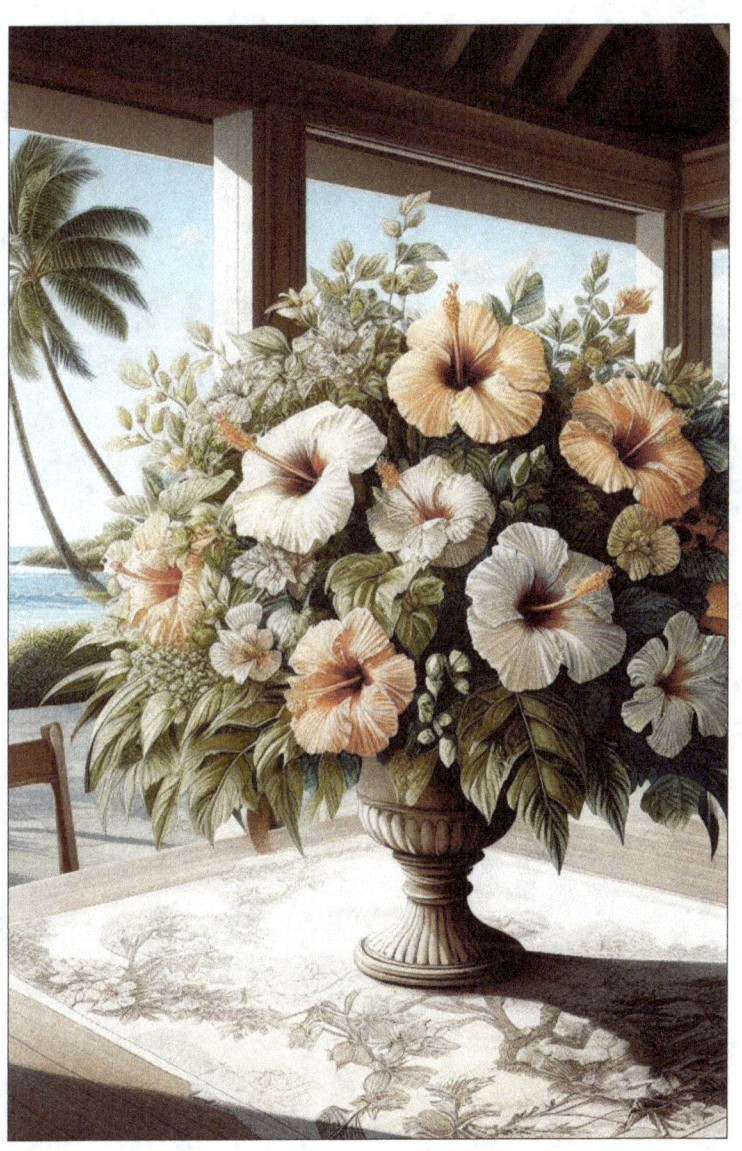

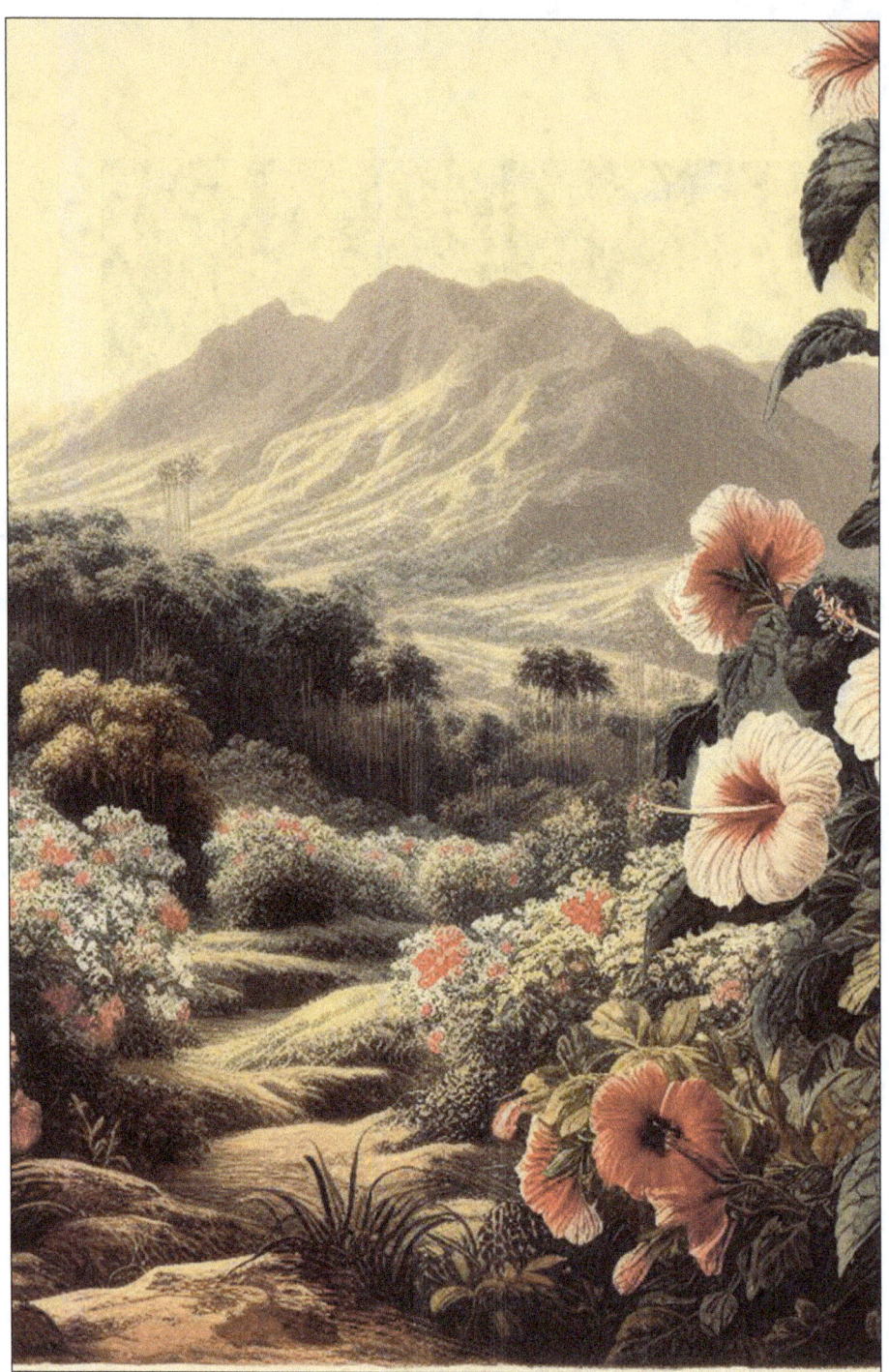

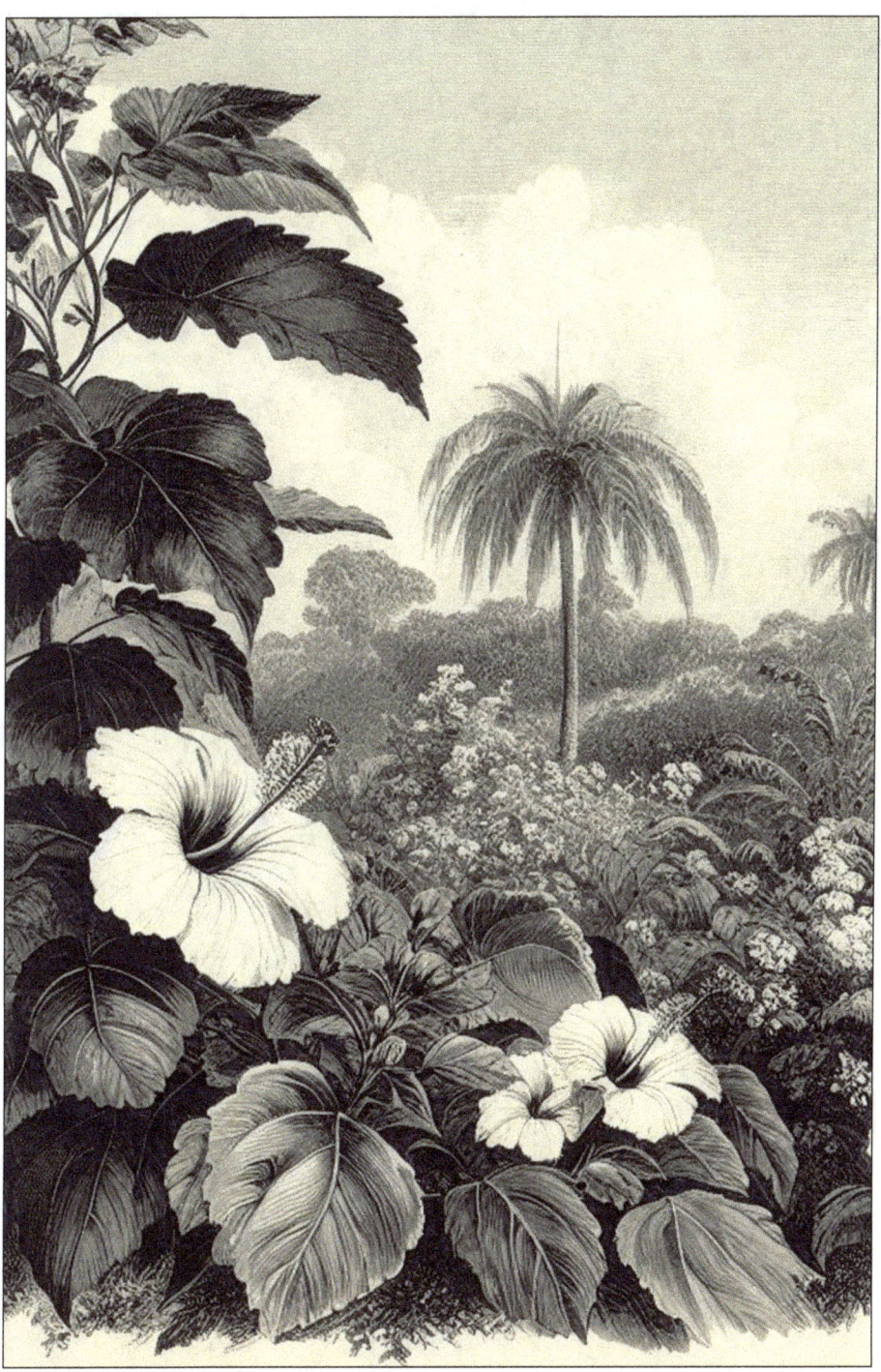

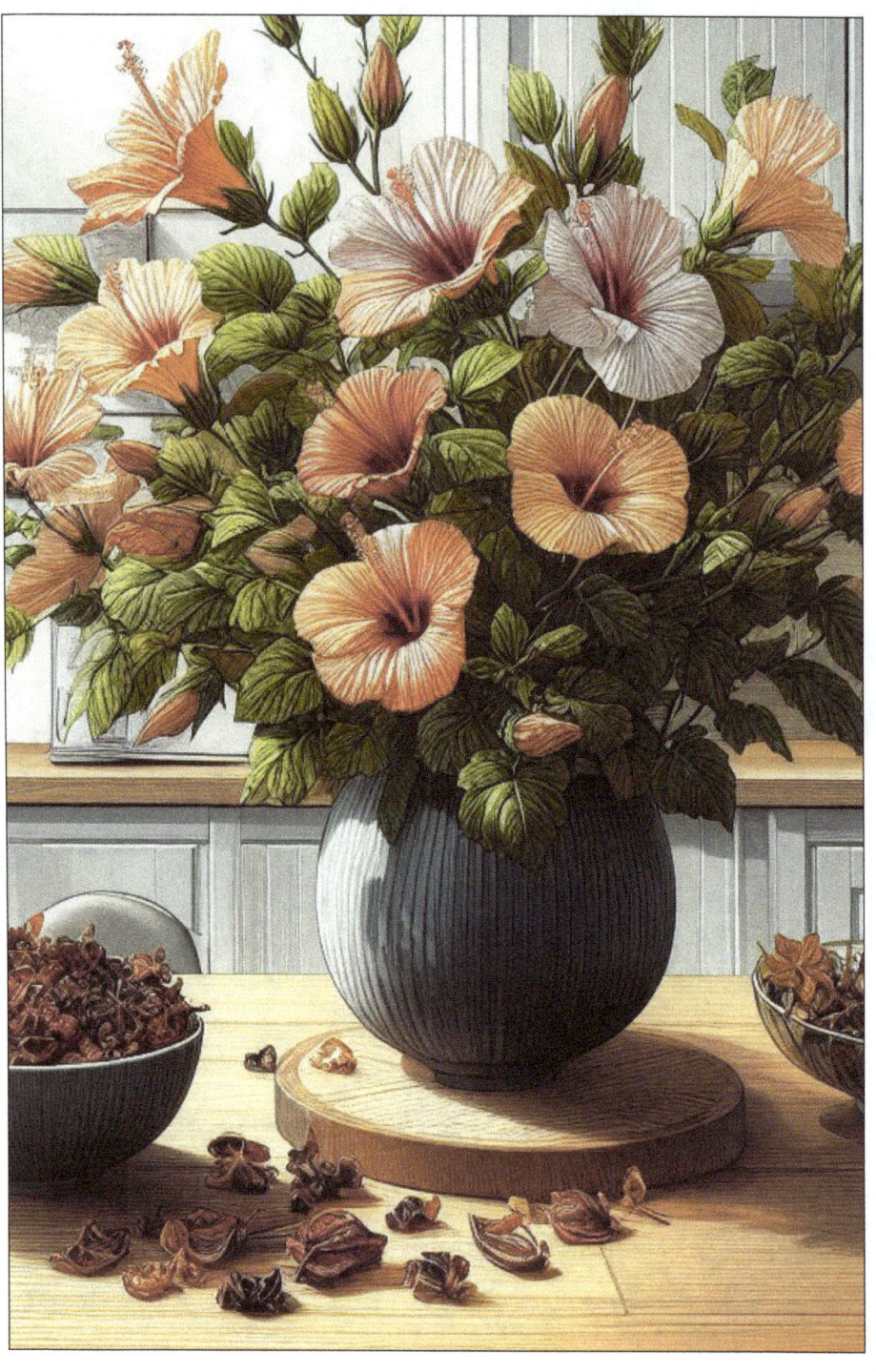

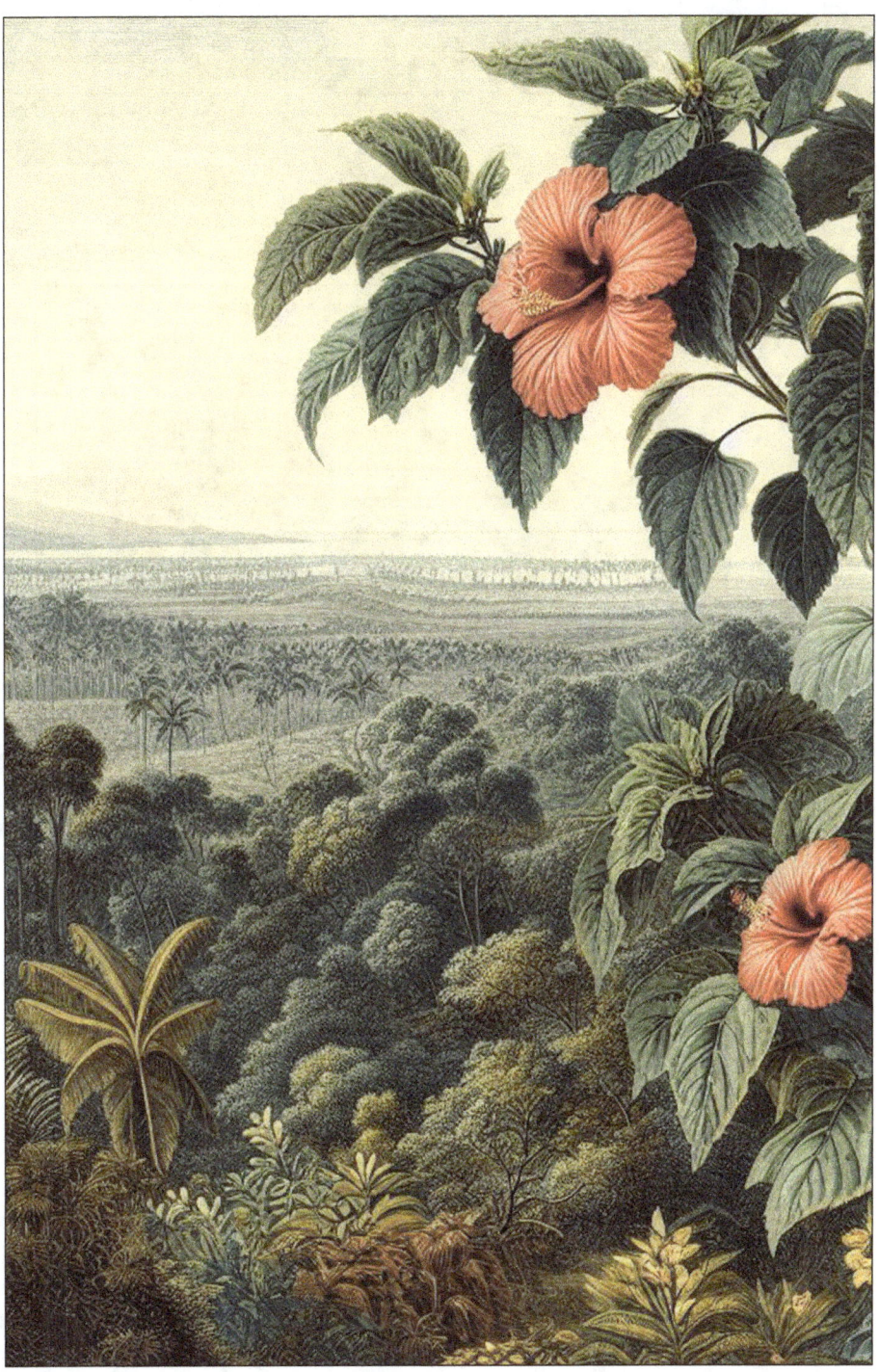

# Drinks

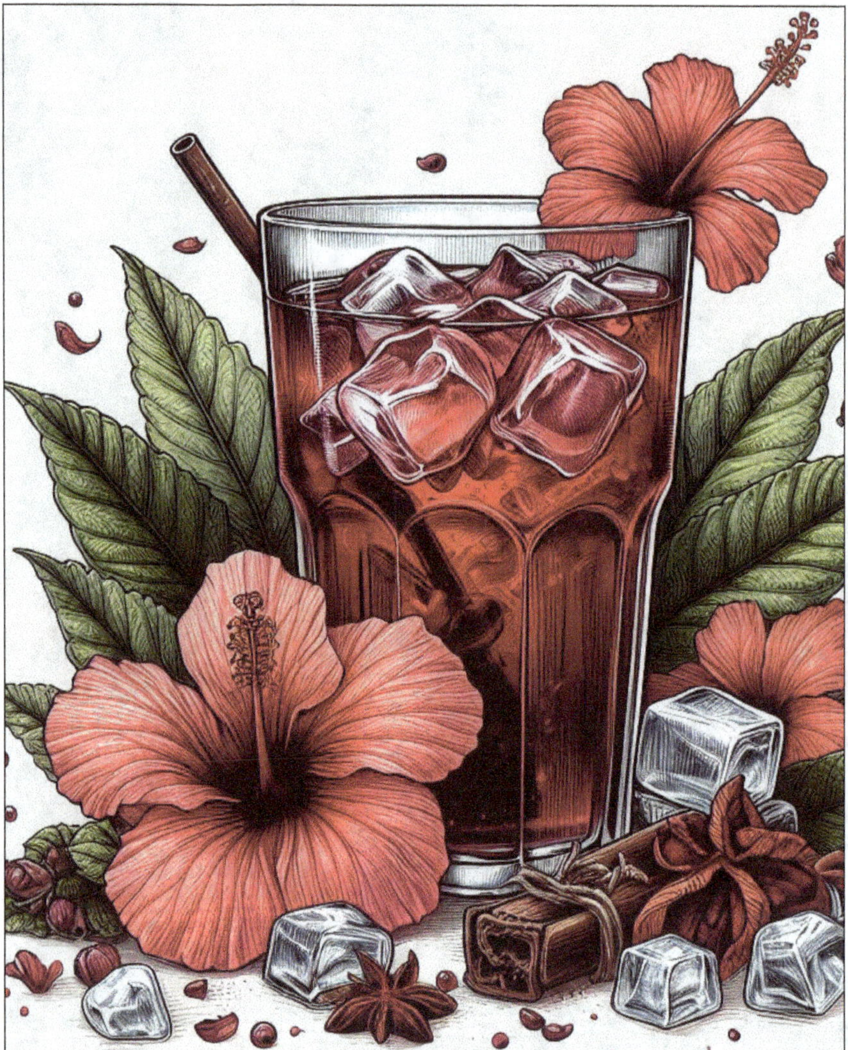

# Classic Hibiscus Iced Tea: A Refreshing Floral Infusion

Hibiscus iced tea is a vibrant and refreshing beverage that combines the tart and floral notes of hibiscus flowers with the crispness of iced tea. This classic recipe is not only visually stunning with its deep red hue but also boasts a delightful flavor profile that is both tangy and slightly sweet. Perfect for hot summer days or any time you crave a revitalizing drink, this hibiscus iced tea is easy to prepare and sure to become a favorite.

## Tips:
1. Experiment with different tea varieties to find your preferred blend. Black tea complements the hibiscus well, but green tea or herbal teas can also work.

2. Adjust the sweetness to your liking. Some may prefer a more tart flavor, while others enjoy a sweeter profile.

3. For an extra touch, consider adding a splash of sparkling water for effervescence.

## Ingredients:
- 1/2 cup dried hibiscus petals
- 4 cups water
- 3-4 black tea bags (or your favorite tea variety)
- 1/4 cup honey or sweetener of your choice (adjust to taste)
- Ice cubes
- Lemon slices and mint leaves for garnish

## Instructions:

1. Infuse the Hibiscus:
  - In a saucepan, bring 4 cups of water to a boil. Once boiling, add the dried hibiscus petals to the water.
  - Reduce the heat to low and let the hibiscus steep for 10-15 minutes. This process allows the water to absorb the vibrant color and tangy flavor of the hibiscus.

2. Brew the Tea:
  - Add the black tea bags to the hibiscus-infused water. Let it steep for an additional 5-7 minutes, adjusting the time based on your desired tea strength.

3. Sweeten to Taste:
  - While the tea is still warm, stir in honey or your preferred sweetener. Start with 1/4 cup and adjust according to your sweetness preference. The floral notes of the hibiscus pair wonderfully with a touch of sweetness.

4. Strain and Chill:
  - Remove the tea bags and strain the hibiscus tea to remove the petals. Allow the tea to cool to room temperature.

5. Refrigerate:
  - Transfer the tea to the refrigerator and let it chill for at least 2 hours. Chilling allows the flavors to meld, resulting in a more harmonious taste.

6. Serve Over Ice:
  - Once thoroughly chilled, fill glasses with ice cubes and pour the hibiscus iced tea over the ice.

7. Garnish and Enjoy:
  - Garnish each glass with a slice of lemon and a few fresh mint leaves for a burst of freshness. Stir gently and enjoy your classic hibiscus iced tea.

# Hibiscus Lemonade: A Zesty Floral Twist to a Summertime Classic

Hibiscus lemonade is a captivating variation of the timeless summer favorite, adding a burst of color and a delightful floral note to the classic citrusy drink. This recipe combines the tartness of lemons with the vibrant, tangy flavor of hibiscus petals, creating a refreshing beverage that not only quenches your thirst but also invigorates your senses. Perfect for hot days, gatherings, or whenever you want to elevate your lemonade experience.

## Tips:
1. Adjust the sugar and water ratios to suit your taste preferences. If you prefer a sweeter lemonade, increase the sugar content accordingly.

2. Experiment with the hibiscus concentration to find your desired level of floral intensity.

3. For a sparkling version, add a splash of sparkling water or soda just before serving.

## Ingredients:
- 1/2 cup dried hibiscus petals
- 1 cup hot water
- 1 cup freshly squeezed lemon juice (approximately 6-8 lemons)
- 1 cup granulated sugar
- 4 cups cold water
- Ice cubes
- Lemon slices and hibiscus flowers for garnish

## Instructions:

1. Hibiscus Infusion:
   - In a heatproof bowl, pour 1 cup of hot water over the dried hibiscus petals. Let it steep for 15-20 minutes, allowing the water to absorb the vibrant color and tangy flavor of the hibiscus.

2. Sweeten the Hibiscus Infusion:
   - While the hibiscus is steeping, dissolve the sugar in 1 cup of hot water, creating a simple syrup. Stir until the sugar is completely dissolved.

3. Strain and Cool:
   - Strain the hibiscus infusion to remove the petals, allowing the liquid to cool to room temperature.

4. Lemon Juice:
   - Squeeze enough lemons to yield 1 cup of fresh lemon juice. This ensures a zesty and authentic lemonade flavor.

5. Combine Ingredients:
   - In a large pitcher, combine the hibiscus infusion, lemon juice, and simple syrup. Stir well to blend the flavors.

6. Add Cold Water:
   - Pour 4 cups of cold water into the pitcher, adjusting to your preferred level of sweetness. Stir until well mixed.

7. Chill:
   - Refrigerate the hibiscus lemonade for at least 2 hours to allow the flavors to meld and intensify.

8. Serve Over Ice:
   - Fill glasses with ice cubes and pour the chilled hibiscus lemonade over the ice.

# Hibiscus Mint Limeade: A Burst of Refreshing Tropical Flavors

Hibiscus mint limeade is a tantalizing beverage that combines the bold floral notes of hibiscus with the crispness of fresh lime and the invigorating aroma of mint. This exotic twist on classic limeade not only offers a visually stunning drink but also provides a harmonious blend of sweet, tart, and herbal flavors. Perfect for warm days or as a unique addition to your beverage repertoire, this hibiscus mint limeade is an irresistible journey for your taste buds.

**Tips:**
1. Adjust the sugar and water ratios to suit your taste preferences. If you prefer a sweeter limeade, increase the sugar content accordingly.

2. For an extra burst of freshness, muddle a few mint leaves in the glass before pouring the limeade.

3. Experiment with the hibiscus concentration for varying levels of floral intensity.

**Ingredients:**

- 1/2 cup dried hibiscus petals
- 1 cup fresh mint leaves
- 1 cup hot water
- 1 cup freshly squeezed lime juice (about 8-10 limes)
- 1 cup granulated sugar
- 4 cups cold water
- Ice cubes
- Lime slices and mint sprigs for garnish

**Instructions:**

1. Hibiscus Mint Infusion:
   - In a heatproof bowl, pour 1 cup of hot water over the dried hibiscus petals and fresh mint leaves. Allow the mixture to steep for 15-20 minutes, letting the water absorb the vibrant colors and aromatic essence.

2. Sweeten the Infusion:
   - While the hibiscus mint infusion is steeping, dissolve the sugar in 1 cup of hot water, creating a mint-infused simple syrup. Stir until the sugar is completely dissolved.

3. Strain and Cool:
   - Strain the hibiscus mint infusion to remove the petals and mint leaves, allowing the liquid to cool to room temperature.

4. Lime Juice:
   - Squeeze enough limes to yield 1 cup of fresh lime juice. This ensures a zesty and authentic limeade flavor.

5. Combine Ingredients:
   - In a large pitcher, combine the hibiscus mint infusion, lime juice, and mint-infused simple syrup. Stir well to ensure a uniform distribution of flavors.

6. Add Cold Water:
   - Pour 4 cups of cold water into the pitcher, adjusting to your preferred level of sweetness. Stir until well mixed.

7. Chill:
   - Refrigerate the hibiscus mint limeade for at least 2 hours to allow the flavors to meld and intensify. Fill glasses with ice cubes and pour the chilled hibiscus mint limeade over the ice.

8. Garnish and Enjoy!

## Sparkling Hibiscus Water: Effervescent Elegance in Every Sip

Sparkling hibiscus water is a fizzy and elegant beverage that infuses the vibrant and tangy essence of hibiscus petals with the effervescence of sparkling water. This effervescent delight is not only visually stunning but also offers a refreshing and sophisticated alternative to plain sparkling water. With its vivid hue and floral undertones, this sparkling hibiscus water is a simple yet enchanting way to elevate your hydration experience.

### Tips:
1. Experiment with different levels of sweetness to find the perfect balance for your taste buds.

2. For a festive touch, consider serving in a stemmed glass with a slice of citrus on the rim.

3. Adjust the hibiscus concentration based on your preference for a stronger or milder floral flavor.

### Ingredients:
- 1/4 cup dried hibiscus petals
- 1 cup hot water
- Sparkling water (chilled)
- Ice cubes
- Optional: Sweetener of choice (agave syrup, honey, or sugar)
- Optional: Lemon or orange slices for garnish

### Instructions:

1. Hibiscus Infusion:
   - Steep 1/4 cup of dried hibiscus petals in 1 cup of hot water for 10-15 minutes, allowing the water to absorb the vibrant color and tangy flavor.

2. Strain and Cool:
   - Strain the hibiscus infusion to remove the petals and let it cool to room temperature. Optionally, sweeten the infusion to your taste preference.

3. Assemble the Drink:
   - In a glass, combine the hibiscus infusion with chilled sparkling water. Adjust the ratio based on your desired strength of flavor.

4. Add Ice:
   - Drop a few ice cubes into the glass to keep the drink cool and refreshing.

5. Garnish (Optional):
   - Garnish with slices of lemon or orange for an extra citrusy twist. Stir gently.

6. Enjoy:
   - Sip and savor the effervescence and floral notes of your sparkling hibiscus water.

# Hibiscus Ginger Ale: A Spicy Floral Fusion for a Zesty Delight

Hibiscus ginger ale is a tantalizing beverage that marries the bold, floral notes of hibiscus with the warm and spicy kick of ginger. This effervescent concoction is not only visually striking with its vibrant color but also offers a delightful fusion of flavors that dance on your palate. Perfect for those who crave a zesty and unique refreshment, hibiscus ginger ale is an invigorating choice that brings together the best of floral and spicy elements.

**Tips:**
1. Adjust the ginger level based on your preference for a milder or spicier kick.

2. Experiment with different varieties of ginger ale for unique flavor profiles.

3. For a fizzy touch, top off each glass with a splash of sparkling water.

**Ingredients:**

- 1/4 cup dried hibiscus petals
- 1 cup hot water
- 1 tablespoon grated fresh ginger
- 1 cup granulated sugar
- 4 cups cold ginger ale
- Ice cubes
- Optional: Lemon or lime slices for garnish

**Instructions:**

1. Hibiscus Infusion:
   - Steep 1/4 cup of dried hibiscus petals in 1 cup of hot water for 10-15 minutes, allowing the water to absorb the vivid color and tangy flavor of the hibiscus.

2. Strain and Cool:
   - Strain the hibiscus infusion to remove the petals, letting it cool to room temperature. Optionally, sweeten the infusion to your taste preference.

3. Ginger Simple Syrup:
   - In a small saucepan, combine grated ginger, sugar, and 1 cup of water. Simmer over medium heat until the sugar dissolves and the ginger infuses into a simple syrup. Allow it to cool.

4. Combine Ingredients:
   - In a large pitcher, mix the hibiscus infusion with the ginger simple syrup. Stir well to blend the flavors.

5. Add Ginger Ale:
   - Pour 4 cups of cold ginger ale into the pitcher, adjusting to your preferred level of sweetness. Stir until well mixed.

6. Chill:
   - Refrigerate the hibiscus ginger ale for at least 1-2 hours to enhance the flavors.

7. Serve Over Ice:
   - Fill glasses with ice cubes and pour the chilled hibiscus ginger ale over the ice.

8. Garnish (Optional):
   - Garnish with slices of lemon or lime for an extra citrusy touch. Stir gently.

9. Enjoy!

## Hibiscus Arnold Palmer: A Floral Twist to the Classic Half and Half Refreshment

The Hibiscus Arnold Palmer is a captivating variation of the classic "Half and Half," combining the timeless duo of iced tea and lemonade with the vibrant and tangy essence of hibiscus petals. This delightful beverage not only refreshes your palate with the briskness of tea and the zing of lemonade but also introduces a unique floral note for an extra layer of sophistication. Whether enjoyed on a warm day or as a flavorful companion to meals, the Hibiscus Arnold Palmer is a refreshing and visually appealing choice.

**Tips:**
1. Experiment with tea varieties and adjust sugar levels based on preference.

2. For a sparkling version, add a splash of sparkling water before serving.

3. Bitters Experimentation: Feel free to experiment with different types of bitters. Some variations, like grapefruit or orange bitters, can complement the citrusy notes in the drink.

**Variations:**

**Herbal Fusion Arnold Palmer:**
Experiment with herbal infusions. Add a bag of chamomile, lavender, or lemongrass tea to the hibiscus mix for a soothing and aromatic variation.

**Spiced Arnold Palmer:**
Sprinkle a pinch of cinnamon or a few cloves into the hibiscus tea for a warm and spiced flavor profile.

**Ingredients:**

- 1/4 cup dried hibiscus petals
- 1 cup hot water
- 3-4 black tea bags
- 1/2 cup freshly squeezed lemon juice
- 1/4 cup granulated sugar
- 4 cups cold water
- Ice cubes
- Lemon slices and hibiscus flowers for garnish

**Instructions:**

1. Steep hibiscus petals in hot water for 10-15 minutes and strain.

2. Sweeten the hibiscus infusion and combine with lemon juice in a pitcher.

3. Brew black tea separately, let it cool, and add it to the pitcher.

4. Pour in cold water, adjusting sweetness to taste. Stir well.

5. Chill for at least 2 hours and serve over ice.

6. Garnish with lemon slices and hibiscus flowers.

7. Enjoy the vibrant combination of tea, lemonade, and hibiscus.

# Hibiscus Agua Fresca: A Refreshing Floral Quencher

Hibiscus Agua Fresca is a revitalizing beverage that showcases the vibrant and tangy flavors of hibiscus petals in a light and hydrating form. This traditional Mexican drink combines the tartness of hibiscus with a touch of sweetness, creating a thirst-quenching experience that is perfect for warm days or as a delightful accompaniment to your meals. Simple yet bursting with flavor, Hibiscus Agua Fresca is a refreshing choice for those seeking a floral and invigorating drink.

## Tips:
1. Experiment with the sugar levels to achieve your preferred balance of sweetness and tartness.

2. For a fizzy version, add a splash of sparkling water just before serving.

3. Customize with additional citrus slices or herbs for a personalized touch.

## Variations:

**Ginger Spice Infusion:**
Add a bit of freshly grated ginger for a spicy kick that complements the tartness of hibiscus.

**Pineapple Hibiscus Splash:**
Mix in pineapple juice or add chunks of fresh pineapple for a tropical and sweet twist.

## Ingredients:
- 1/2 cup dried hibiscus petals
- 4 cups water
- 1/3 cup granulated sugar (adjust to taste)
- Ice cubes
- Fresh mint leaves for garnish
- Optional: Slices of orange or lime for extra citrusy notes

## Instructions:

1. **Hibiscus Infusion:**
   - Steep 1/2 cup of dried hibiscus petals in 4 cups of hot water for 15-20 minutes. Allow the water to absorb the vivid color and tangy flavor of the hibiscus.

2. **Sweeten to Taste:**
   - While the hibiscus is steeping, dissolve sugar in the infusion. Adjust the sweetness to your preference.

3. **Strain and Cool:**
   - Strain the hibiscus infusion to remove the petals and let it cool to room temperature.

4. **Chill:**
   - Refrigerate the hibiscus agua fresca for at least 1-2 hours to enhance the flavors.

5. **Serve Over Ice:**
   - Fill glasses with ice cubes and pour the chilled hibiscus agua fresca over the ice.

6. **Garnish (Optional):**
   - Garnish with fresh mint leaves and slices of orange or lime for an extra burst of flavor.

7. **Enjoy:**
   - Sip and savor the refreshing and floral notes of the Hibiscus Agua Fresca.

# Hibiscus Blueberry Sparkler: A Burst of Berry-Floral Bliss

The Hibiscus Blueberry Sparkler is a dazzling beverage that fuses the vibrant and tangy notes of hibiscus with the sweetness of blueberries, all elevated by the effervescence of sparkling water. This sparkling concoction is not only visually stunning but also offers a delightful symphony of flavors that dance on your taste buds. Perfect for celebrations or as a unique and refreshing treat, the Hibiscus Blueberry Sparkler is a delightful way to elevate your sparkling beverage experience.

---

### Tips:
1. Experiment with the sweetness level by adjusting the amount of honey or agave syrup.

2. For a visually striking presentation, use clear glasses to showcase the vibrant colors.

3. Try adding a splash of citrus juice for an extra layer of complexity.

---

### Ingredients:
- 1/4 cup dried hibiscus petals
- 1 cup hot water
- 1/2 cup fresh blueberries
- 1-2 tablespoons honey or agave syrup
- Sparkling water
- Ice cubes
- Blueberries and hibiscus flowers for garnish

---

### Instructions:

1. Hibiscus Blueberry Infusion:
   - Steep hibiscus petals in hot water for 15-20 minutes. Strain and sweeten with honey or agave syrup.

2. Blueberry Puree:
   - Blend fresh blueberries until smooth. Strain for a smoother consistency.

3. Combine Ingredients:
   - Mix hibiscus infusion with blueberry puree in a pitcher.

4. Add Sparkling Water:
   - Pour chilled sparkling water just before serving. Adjust to your desired effervescence.

5. Chill:
   - Refrigerate for 1-2 hours to enhance flavors.

6. Serve Over Ice:
   - Pour over ice in glasses.

7. Garnish:
   - Add fresh blueberries and hibiscus flowers for an elegant touch.

8. Enjoy:
   - Savor the delightful combination of hibiscus, blueberries, and sparkling effervescence.

# Coconut Hibiscus Cooler: Tropical Refreshment

The Coconut Hibiscus Cooler is more than just a refreshing drink; it's a tropical symphony of flavors with potential health benefits. This delightful beverage combines the vibrant tang of hibiscus petals with the tropical essence of coconut water, offering a unique and hydrating experience.

## Tips:
1. Adjust sweetness to your liking.

2. Experiment with coconut milk for a creamier texture.

3. For an extra chill, freeze coconut water into ice cubes.

## Potential Health Benefits:

**1. Rich in Antioxidants:** Hibiscus is renowned for its high antioxidant content, which may help combat oxidative stress and inflammation in the body.

**2. Hydration Boost:** Coconut water is a natural source of electrolytes, making it an excellent choice for rehydration. It's low in calories and provides essential minerals.

**3. Heart Health:** Some studies suggest that hibiscus may contribute to heart health by helping to lower blood pressure and cholesterol levels.

**4. Immune Support:** Both hibiscus and coconut water contain vitamins and minerals that can support a healthy immune system.

**5. Skin Benefits:** Antioxidants in hibiscus may promote skin health, while coconut water's hydrating properties contribute to a radiant complexion.

## Ingredients:

- 1/4 cup dried hibiscus petals
- 1 cup hot water
- 1/2 cup coconut water
- 1-2 tablespoons agave syrup (adjust to taste)
- Ice cubes
- Hibiscus flowers and coconut slices for garnish

## Instructions:

1. Hibiscus Infusion:
   - Steep hibiscus petals in hot water for 15-20 minutes. Strain and let it cool.

2. Combine Ingredients:
   - In a glass, mix the hibiscus infusion with coconut water.

3. Sweeten:
   - Add agave syrup to achieve your preferred level of sweetness.

4. Chill:
   - Refrigerate for at least 1 hour to enhance flavors.

5. Serve Over Ice:
   - Pour over ice in a glass.

6. Garnish:
   - Garnish with hibiscus flowers and coconut slices.

7. Enjoy:
   - Sip and enjoy the tropical fusion of coconut and hibiscus.

## Hibiscus and Basil Lemon Fizz: A Refreshing Herbal Elixir

The Hibiscus and Basil Lemon Fizz is a tantalizing blend of floral hibiscus, aromatic basil, and zesty lemon, creating a refreshing herbal elixir. This effervescent drink is not only visually striking but also bursts with unique flavors.

---

### Tips:
1. Experiment with Herb Infusion: Try varying the basil infusion time for a more pronounced or subtle herbal essence.

2. Adjust Sweetness: Tailor the sweetness level by adjusting the amount of honey or agave syrup to suit your taste preferences.

3. Temperature Matters: For the most refreshing experience, ensure your sparkling water is well-chilled before adding to the mix.

4. Play with Presentation: Impress your guests by serving in clear glasses to showcase the vibrant colors. Add a basil leaf or two on top for an extra touch.

---

### Variations;

**Chili Basil Spice:**
For those who enjoy a bit of heat, add a tiny pinch of chili powder or a slice of fresh chili for a spicy kick.

**Honey Basil Serenity:**
Drizzle a bit of honey into the drink to add a natural sweetness that complements the tartness of the hibiscus and the herbal notes of basil.

### Ingredients:

- 1/4 cup dried hibiscus petals
- 1 cup hot water
- Handful of fresh basil leaves
- 1/2 cup freshly squeezed lemon juice
- 1-2 tablespoons honey or agave syrup (adjust to taste)
- Sparkling water (chilled)
- Ice cubes
- Basil leaves and lemon slices for garnish

### Instructions:

1. Hibiscus Basil Infusion:
   - Steep hibiscus petals in hot water for 15-20 minutes. Add fresh basil leaves during the last 5 minutes. Strain.

2. Sweeten:
   - Mix in honey or agave syrup to your preferred sweetness level.

3. Citrusy Twist:
   - Combine the hibiscus basil infusion with freshly squeezed lemon juice for a zesty kick.

4. Fizz it Up:
   - Just before serving, pour the mixture over ice and top it off with chilled sparkling water.

5. Garnish:
   - Garnish with basil leaves and lemon slices for a visually appealing finish.

6. Enjoy:
   - Sip and revel in the herbal and citrusy delight of your Hibiscus and Basil Lemon Fizz.

# Hibiscus Rosemary Spritzer: A Herbal Infusion with Sparkle

The Hibiscus Rosemary Spritzer is a delightful marriage of floral hibiscus and fragrant rosemary, creating a herbal infusion with a sparkling twist. This spritzer is not only a feast for the taste buds but also a visual treat, making it a perfect beverage for any occasion.

## Tips:

1. Herb Infusion Intensity: Adjust the infusion time for rosemary to control the herbal intensity. Steep longer for a bolder flavor.

2. Balance the Sweetness: Experiment with the sweetness level by altering the amount of honey or agave syrup. Find the perfect balance for your palate.

3. Presentation Matters: Serve in tall glasses with a rosemary sprig as a stirrer for an elegant presentation.

4. Chill Sparkling Water: Ensure your sparkling water is well-chilled to maintain the refreshing effervescence of the spritzer.

## Ingredients:

- 1/4 cup dried hibiscus petals
- 1 cup hot water
- Fresh rosemary sprigs
- 1/2 cup sparkling water (chilled)
- 1-2 tablespoons honey or agave syrup (adjust to taste)
- Ice cubes
- Rosemary sprigs and hibiscus petals for garnish

## Instructions:

1. Hibiscus Rosemary Infusion:
   - Steep hibiscus petals in hot water for 15-20 minutes. Add fresh rosemary sprigs during the last 5 minutes. Strain.

2. Sweeten:
   - Mix in honey or agave syrup to your desired level of sweetness.

3. Fizz it Up:
   - Pour the hibiscus rosemary infusion over ice and top it off with chilled sparkling water.

4. Garnish:
   - Garnish with rosemary sprigs and hibiscus petals for a visually appealing touch.

5. Enjoy:
   - Sip and savor the harmonious blend of hibiscus and rosemary in this effervescent spritzer.

# Spiced Hibiscus Chai: A Flavorful Fusion of Spice and Floral

The Spiced Hibiscus Chai is a symphony of flavors, combining the floral notes of hibiscus with the warmth of chai spices. This aromatic infusion is not only a comforting beverage but also a delightful journey for your senses.

---

## Tips:
1. Play with Spice Intensity: Adjust the quantity of cloves, cinnamon, and ginger to suit your spice preference.

2. Milk Choice: Experiment with different types of milk, such as dairy, almond, or oat, for varied creaminess.

3. Control Sweetness: Customize the sweetness by varying the amount of honey or agave syrup. Taste and adjust accordingly.

4. Presentation Detail: Serve in your favorite mug and garnish with a sprinkle of ground cinnamon for an added visual and aromatic touch.

---

## Variations:

### Rosemary Citrus Fusion:
Take your Spiced Hibiscus Chai to a new level by incorporating the unexpected twist of fresh rosemary and citrus zest. The herbal notes of rosemary and the citrusy brightness create a unique and refreshing flavor profile.

### Black Pepper Pineapple Surprise:
Add a surprising kick to your Spiced Hibiscus Chai by introducing freshly ground black pepper and the sweet tanginess of pineapple. This oddball combination provides a perfect balance of heat, spice, and tropical sweetness.

---

## Ingredients:

- 1/4 cup dried hibiscus petals
- 1 cup hot water
- 2 black tea bags
- 1 cinnamon stick
- 3-4 whole cloves
- 1-inch fresh ginger, sliced
- 1-2 tablespoons honey or agave syrup (adjust to taste)
- 1/2 cup milk (dairy or plant-based)
- Optional: Ground cinnamon for garnish

---

## Instructions:

1. Hibiscus Chai Infusion:
   - Steep hibiscus petals and black tea bags in hot water for 15-20 minutes. Add cinnamon stick, cloves, and sliced ginger. Strain.

2. Sweeten and Add Milk:
   - Mix in honey or agave syrup to your preferred sweetness. Add milk to the hibiscus chai infusion and warm the mixture.

3. Strain and Serve:
   - Strain the spiced hibiscus chai into a cup. Optionally, sprinkle with ground cinnamon for an extra layer of spice.

4. Enjoy:
   - Sip and relish the warm and spiced fusion of hibiscus and chai.

# Hibiscus Green Tea Blend: A Refreshing Harmony of Floral and Green

The Hibiscus Green Tea Blend is a refreshing concoction that brings together the tartness of hibiscus with the crispness of green tea. This vibrant blend is not only a feast for the taste buds but also a revitalizing treat for any time of the day.

## Tips:
1. Experiment with Tea Types: Explore different varieties of green tea to find the one that complements the hibiscus flavor best.

2. Temperature Control: Adjust the water temperature for green tea to avoid bitterness. Aim for around 175°F (80°C).

3. Customize Sweetness: Tailor the sweetness to your liking by adjusting the amount of honey or agave syrup.

4. Minty Freshness: If you enjoy minty notes, add fresh mint leaves for an extra layer of flavor.

## Ingredients:

- 1/4 cup dried hibiscus petals
- 1 cup hot water
- 1 green tea bag
- 1-2 tablespoons honey or agave syrup (adjust to taste)
- Optional: Mint leaves for freshness
- Ice cubes

## Instructions:

1. Hibiscus Green Tea Infusion:
   - Steep hibiscus petals and a green tea bag in hot water for 5-7 minutes. Strain.

2. Sweeten:
   - Mix in honey or agave syrup to your preferred level of sweetness.

3. Chill:
   - Allow the hibiscus green tea infusion to cool, or refrigerate for a faster chill.

4. Serve Over Ice:
   - Pour the chilled blend over ice cubes for a refreshing twist.

5. Optional Freshness:
   - Enhance with mint leaves for a burst of freshness.

6. Enjoy:
   - Sip and enjoy the revitalizing blend of hibiscus and green tea.

# Hibiscus Pineapple Punch: Tropical Bliss in a Glass

The Hibiscus Pineapple Punch is a tropical escape in a glass, marrying the tartness of hibiscus with the sweet and tangy notes of pineapple. This punch is not only a visual delight but also a refreshing and exotic treat for your taste buds.

## Tips:
1. Experiment with Ratios: Adjust the ratio of hibiscus infusion to pineapple juice to find the perfect balance for your taste.

2. Temperature Consideration: Ensure the sparkling water is well-chilled to maintain the punch's refreshing fizz.

3. Garnish Creatively: Play with different garnishes like a pineapple wedge on the rim or a sprig of mint for an extra touch of elegance.

4. Serve in Style: Use a transparent pitcher or glass to showcase the vibrant colors of the punch.

## Ingredients:
- 1/4 cup dried hibiscus petals
- 1 cup hot water
- 1/2 cup pineapple juice
- 1-2 tablespoons honey or agave syrup (adjust to taste)
- 1 cup sparkling water (chilled)
- Ice cubes
- Pineapple slices and mint leaves for garnish

## Instructions:

1. Hibiscus Infusion:
   - Steep hibiscus petals in hot water for 15-20 minutes. Strain to create a vibrant hibiscus infusion.

2. Sweeten and Chill:
   - Mix in honey or agave syrup to your desired sweetness. Allow the hibiscus infusion to cool or refrigerate for a faster chill.

3. Pineapple Addition:
   - Combine the hibiscus infusion with pineapple juice for a tropical twist.

4. Fizz it Up:
   - Just before serving, add chilled sparkling water to the punch for a fizzy burst.

5. Serve Over Ice:
   - Pour the Hibiscus Pineapple Punch over ice cubes for a refreshing feel.

6. Garnish:
   - Garnish with pineapple slices and mint leaves to elevate the visual appeal.

7. Enjoy:
   - Sip and bask in the tropical bliss of this delightful punch.

# Hibiscus Cranberry Virgin Cocktail with a Quirky Twist

The Hibiscus Cranberry Virgin Cocktail surprises your taste buds with an unexpected hint of balsamic vinegar, adding a unique twist to the classic combination of hibiscus and cranberry. This refreshing and quirky mocktail is a conversation starter at any gathering.

## Tips:
1. Balsamic Vinegar Quality: Choose a high-quality balsamic vinegar to ensure a rich and nuanced flavor.

2. Adjust Sweetness: Fine-tune the sweetness by experimenting with the amount of honey or agave syrup.

3. Presentation Flair: Serve in mocktail glasses with a hibiscus petal on top for a visually appealing presentation.

4. Citrus Zest Upgrade: Enhance the orange garnish by expressing the citrus oils over the mocktail for an extra burst of aroma.

## Ingredients:

- 1/4 cup dried hibiscus petals
- 1 cup hot water
- 1/2 cup cranberry juice
- 1-2 tablespoons honey or agave syrup (adjust to taste)
- 1/2 teaspoon balsamic vinegar (the quirky twist!)
- Sparkling water (chilled)
- Ice cubes
- Orange slices for garnish

## Instructions:

1. Hibiscus Infusion:
   - Steep hibiscus petals in hot water for 15-20 minutes. Strain to create a vibrant hibiscus infusion.

2. Sweeten and Chill:
   - Mix in honey or agave syrup to achieve your desired sweetness. Allow the hibiscus infusion to cool or refrigerate for a faster chill.

3. Cranberry Blend:
   - Combine the hibiscus infusion with cranberry juice for a tangy and floral base.

4. Balsamic Vinegar Twist:
   - Add a quirky twist with a half teaspoon of balsamic vinegar, enhancing the complexity of flavors.

5. Fizz it Up:
   - Just before serving, top off the mocktail with chilled sparkling water for a lively effervescence.

6. Serve Over Ice:
   - Pour the Hibiscus Cranberry Mocktail over ice cubes.

7. Garnish:
   - Garnish with a slice of orange for a burst of citrusy aroma.

8. Enjoy:
   - Sip and savor the unexpected harmony of hibiscus, cranberry, and the quirky balsamic vinegar twist.

# Smoothies

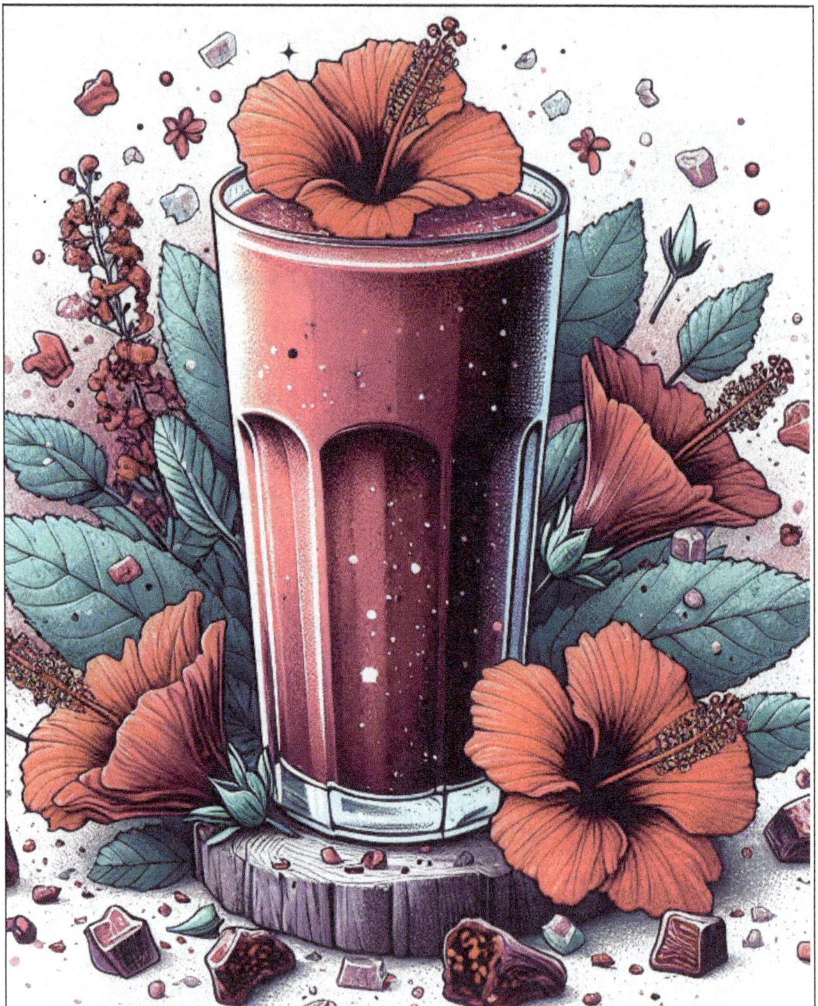

# Tropical Hibiscus Smoothie: A Vibrant Burst of Exotic Flavors

The Tropical Hibiscus Smoothie invites you on a journey to the tropics with the infusion of hibiscus, pineapple, mango, and coconut. This smoothie is not only a feast for the taste buds but also a revitalizing treat that brings the essence of a tropical paradise to your glass.

## Tips:
1. Frozen Fruit for Creaminess: Using frozen pineapple and mango chunks adds creaminess and eliminates the need for additional ice.

2. Chia Seeds Boost: For a nutritional boost and added texture, consider incorporating chia seeds into the smoothie.

3. Consistency Adjustment: Adjust the thickness of the smoothie by adding more coconut milk or water, depending on your preference.

4. Garnish Creatively: Garnish with a hibiscus petal or a slice of pineapple on the rim of the glass for a decorative touch.

## Ingredients:

- 1/4 cup dried hibiscus petals
- 1 cup hot water
- 1/2 cup pineapple chunks (fresh or frozen)
- 1/2 cup mango chunks (fresh or frozen)
- 1 banana
- 1/2 cup coconut milk
- Ice cubes
- Optional: Chia seeds for added texture

## Instructions:

1. Hibiscus Infusion:
   - Steep hibiscus petals in hot water for 15-20 minutes. Strain to create a vibrant hibiscus infusion.

2. Blend Tropical Goodness:
   - In a blender, combine the hibiscus infusion with pineapple chunks, mango chunks, banana, and coconut milk. Blend until smooth.

3. Ice and Chia Seeds:
   - Add ice cubes to the blender for a refreshing chill. Optionally, toss in chia seeds for added texture and nutritional benefits.

4. Blend Again:
   - Blend all ingredients until the mixture reaches a smooth and creamy consistency.

5. Pour and Serve:
   - Pour the Tropical Hibiscus Smoothie into glasses and serve immediately.

6. Enjoy:
   - Sip and indulge in the exotic medley of tropical flavors in every refreshing sip.

# Berry Hibiscus Smoothie Bowl: A Colorful Fusion of Berries and Floral Bliss

The Berry Hibiscus Smoothie Bowl is a feast for the senses, combining the tartness of hibiscus with the sweetness of mixed berries. This bowl is not only a treat for the taste buds but also a visual delight, showcasing a colorful array of toppings.

## Tips:
1. Hibiscus as a Base: Let the hibiscus infusion be the star, adjusting the amount of berries to your taste preference.

2. Customize Toppings: Get creative with toppings; choose a mix of textures and flavors like crunchy granola, chewy chia seeds, and the freshness of coconut and berries.

3. Consistency Control: Adjust the thickness of the smoothie by adding more or less Greek yogurt.

4. Personalize Sweetness: Taste the smoothie before adding honey, as the sweetness of the berries and hibiscus might be sufficient.

## Ingredients:

- 1/4 cup dried hibiscus petals
- 1 cup hot water
- 1 cup mixed berries (strawberries, blueberries, raspberries)
- 1 banana
- 1/2 cup Greek yogurt
- 1 tablespoon honey or agave syrup (optional, for sweetness)
- Toppings: Fresh berries, granola, coconut flakes, chia seeds

## Instructions:

1. Hibiscus Infusion:
   - Steep hibiscus petals in hot water for 15-20 minutes. Strain to create a vibrant hibiscus infusion.

2. Blend Berry Goodness:
   - In a blender, combine the hibiscus infusion with mixed berries, banana, Greek yogurt, and honey (if using). Blend until smooth.

3. Pour into a Bowl:
   - Pour the Berry Hibiscus Smoothie into a bowl.

4. Toppings Galore:
   - Top with a generous handful of fresh berries, granola, coconut flakes, and a sprinkle of chia seeds.

5. Enjoy with a Spoon:
   - Dive in with a spoon and relish the burst of flavors and textures in every bite.

# Citrus Hibiscus Bliss Smoothie: A Zesty Floral Delight

The Citrus Hibiscus Bliss Smoothie is a celebration of bright and zesty citrus fruits harmonized with the floral notes of hibiscus. This smoothie is not only a burst of refreshing flavors but also a revitalizing experience that awakens the senses.

## Tips:
1. Adjust Sweetness Naturally: Taste the smoothie before adding honey, as the natural sweetness of citrus and hibiscus might be sufficient.

2. Texture Variation: For added texture, consider blending in a handful of crushed ice or frozen citrus segments.

3. Experiment with Citrus: Feel free to try different citrus fruits like mandarins or blood oranges to customize the flavor profile.

4. Consistency Control: Adjust the thickness of the smoothie by varying the amount of yogurt.

## Ingredients:

- 1/4 cup dried hibiscus petals
- 1 cup hot water
- 1 orange, peeled and segmented
- 1/2 grapefruit, peeled and segmented
- 1 banana
- 1/2 cup plain yogurt
- 1 tablespoon honey or agave syrup (optional, for sweetness)
- Ice cubes

## Instructions:

1. Hibiscus Infusion:
   - Steep hibiscus petals in hot water for 15-20 minutes. Strain to create a vibrant hibiscus infusion.

2. Citrus Burst:
   - In a blender, combine the hibiscus infusion with orange segments, grapefruit segments, banana, yogurt, and honey (if using). Blend until smooth.

3. Chill with Ice:
   - Add ice cubes to the blender and blend again until the smoothie reaches a refreshing and chilled consistency.

4. Pour into a Glass:
   - Pour the Citrus Hibiscus Bliss Smoothie into a glass.

5. Garnish (Optional):
   - Garnish with a slice of orange or a hibiscus petal for a decorative touch.

6. Sip and Enjoy:
   - Sip and revel in the zesty and floral bliss of this refreshing citrus-infused smoothie.

# Hibiscus Peach Passion Smoothie: A Tropical Symphony in a Glass

The Hibiscus Peach Passion Smoothie invites you on a journey to the tropics with the infusion of hibiscus, the sweetness of peaches, and the exotic allure of passion fruit. This smoothie is not only a treat for the taste buds but also a refreshing escape to paradise.

## Tips:
1. Frozen Fruits for Creaminess: Using frozen peach slices enhances the creaminess of the smoothie without the need for additional ice.

2. Passion Fruit Pulp Prep: If using fresh passion fruit, scoop out the pulp and strain the seeds before adding to the blender.

3. Natural Sweetness: The natural sweetness from peaches and passion fruit may be enough; taste before adding sweeteners.

4. Consistency Control: Adjust the thickness of the smoothie by varying the amount of coconut water.

## Ingredients:
- 1/4 cup dried hibiscus petals
- 1 cup hot water
- 1 cup frozen peach slices
- 1/2 cup passion fruit pulp (fresh or frozen)
- 1 banana
- 1/2 cup coconut water
- 1 tablespoon honey or agave syrup (optional, for sweetness)
- Ice cubes

## Instructions:

1. Hibiscus Infusion:
   - Steep hibiscus petals in hot water for 15-20 minutes. Strain to create a vibrant hibiscus infusion.

2. Tropical Fusion:
   - In a blender, combine the hibiscus infusion with frozen peach slices, passion fruit pulp, banana, coconut water, and honey (if using). Blend until smooth.

3. Chill with Ice:
   - Add ice cubes to the blender and blend again until the smoothie reaches a refreshing and chilled consistency.

4. Pour into a Glass:
   - Pour the Hibiscus Peach Passion Smoothie into a glass.

5. Garnish (Optional):
   - Garnish with a slice of peach or a hibiscus petal for a delightful touch.

6. Sip and Enjoy:
   - Sip and savor the tropical symphony of flavors in this luscious and exotic smoothie.

# Minty Watermelon Hibiscus Smoothie: A Cool and Refreshing Fusion

The Minty Watermelon Hibiscus Smoothie is a refreshing blend that combines the hydrating essence of watermelon with the floral notes of hibiscus and a minty kick. This smoothie is not only a treat for the taste buds but also a revitalizing sip on a hot day.

## Tips:
1. Seedless Watermelon: Opt for seedless watermelon to save time on deseeding and ensure a smoother texture.

2. Fresh Mint Impact: Use fresh mint leaves for a vibrant and aromatic minty flavor.

3. Lime Zest Technique: Add an extra layer of citrusy brightness by incorporating a bit of lime zest into the smoothie.

4. Consistency Control: Adjust the thickness of the smoothie by adding more or less ice cubes.

## Ingredients:

- 1/4 cup dried hibiscus petals
- 1 cup hot water
- 2 cups fresh watermelon, cubed and deseeded
- 1/2 cup cucumber, peeled and diced
- Fresh mint leaves (about 10 leaves)
- 1 tablespoon lime juice
- 1 tablespoon honey or agave syrup (optional, for sweetness)
- Ice cubes

## Instructions:

1. Hibiscus Infusion:
   - Steep hibiscus petals in hot water for 15-20 minutes. Strain to create a vibrant hibiscus infusion.

2. Cooling Watermelon Mix:
   - In a blender, combine the hibiscus infusion with fresh watermelon, cucumber, mint leaves, lime juice, and honey (if using). Blend until smooth.

3. Chill with Ice:
   - Add ice cubes to the blender and blend again until the smoothie reaches a cool and slushy consistency.

4. Pour into a Glass:
   - Pour the Minty Watermelon Hibiscus Smoothie into a glass.

5. Garnish (Optional):
   - Garnish with a mint sprig or a watermelon wedge for a touch of freshness.

6. Sip and Enjoy:
   - Sip and revel in the cool and minty embrace of this revitalizing watermelon and hibiscus smoothie.

# Creamy Hibiscus Avocado Smoothie: A Luxurious Fusion of Flavors

The Creamy Hibiscus Avocado Smoothie is a decadent and luscious blend that merges the creamy texture of avocado with the floral notes of hibiscus. This smoothie is not only a treat for the taste buds but also a luxurious experience that adds a touch of elegance to your day.

## Tips:
1. Ripe Avocado is Key: Ensure the avocado is fully ripe for the creamiest texture and optimal flavor.

2. Sweetness Balance: Adjust the sweetness to your liking by experimenting with the amount of honey or agave syrup.

3. Texture Enhancement: For an even creamier consistency, consider using frozen banana slices instead of fresh.

4. Consistency Control: Customize the thickness of the smoothie by adding more or fewer ice cubes.

## Ingredients:
- 1/4 cup dried hibiscus petals
- 1 cup hot water
- 1 ripe avocado, peeled and pitted
- 1 banana
- 1/2 cup Greek yogurt
- 1-2 tablespoons honey or agave syrup (adjust to taste)
- Ice cubes

## Instructions:

1. Hibiscus Infusion:
   - Steep hibiscus petals in hot water for 15-20 minutes. Strain to create a vibrant hibiscus infusion.

2. Creamy Blend:
   - In a blender, combine the hibiscus infusion with ripe avocado, banana, Greek yogurt, and honey (if using). Blend until the mixture is smooth and creamy.

3. Chill with Ice:
   - Add ice cubes to the blender and blend again until the smoothie reaches a luxurious and chilled consistency.

4. Pour into a Glass:
   - Pour the Creamy Hibiscus Avocado Smoothie into a glass.

5. Garnish (Optional):
   - Garnish with a hibiscus petal or a slice of avocado for an elegant touch.

6. Sip and Enjoy:
   - Sip and savor the velvety richness of this indulgent hibiscus and avocado smoothie.

# Hibiscus Banana Berry Blast: A Burst of Berries and Tropical Sweetness

The Hibiscus Banana Berry Blast is a lively and fruity concoction that combines the tropical sweetness of pineapple with the burst of berries and the floral notes of hibiscus. This smoothie is not only a celebration of flavors but also a refreshing sip that transports you to a tropical paradise.

## Tips:

1. Frozen Fruit Boost: Use frozen banana slices and berries for added creaminess and a chill factor.

2. Pineapple Magic: The pineapple chunks add a tropical twist; adjust the quantity based on your preference for sweetness.

3. Natural Sweetness: Taste the smoothie before adding sweeteners, as the natural sugars from the fruits and hibiscus might be sufficient.

4. Consistency Control: Customize the thickness of the smoothie by adding more or fewer ice cubes.

## Ingredients:

- 1/4 cup dried hibiscus petals
- 1 cup hot water
- 1 banana
- 1/2 cup mixed berries (strawberries, blueberries, raspberries)
- 1/2 cup pineapple chunks (fresh or frozen)
- 1 tablespoon honey or agave syrup (optional, for sweetness)
- Ice cubes

## Instructions:

1. Hibiscus Infusion:
   - Steep hibiscus petals in hot water for 15-20 minutes. Strain to create a vibrant hibiscus infusion.

2. Fruity Fusion:
   - In a blender, combine the hibiscus infusion with banana, mixed berries, pineapple chunks, and honey (if using). Blend until the mixture is smooth and bursting with fruity flavors.

3. Chill with Ice:
   - Add ice cubes to the blender and blend again until the smoothie reaches a refreshing and chilled consistency.

4. Pour into a Glass:
   - Pour the Hibiscus Banana Berry Blast into a glass.

5. Garnish (Optional):
   - Garnish with a hibiscus petal or a slice of pineapple for a delightful touch.

6. Sip and Enjoy:
   - Sip and revel in the tropical sweetness and berry explosion of this vibrant hibiscus-infused smoothie.

# Mango Tango Hibiscus Smoothie: A Dance of Tropical Sweetness

The Mango Tango Hibiscus Smoothie is a lively and tropical dance of flavors, blending the sweetness of mango with the floral notes of hibiscus and the creamy touch of coconut. This smoothie is not only a treat for the taste buds but also a refreshing escape to a tropical paradise.

## Tips:
1. Frozen Mango Goodness: Using frozen mango chunks adds a creamy and chill factor to the smoothie.

2. Orange Juice Zest: Choose freshly squeezed orange juice for a burst of citrusy freshness.

3. Coconut Milk Creaminess: Adjust the quantity of coconut milk for your preferred level of creaminess.

4. Natural Sweetness: Taste the smoothie before adding sweeteners, as the natural sugars from the fruits and hibiscus might be sufficient.

## Ingredients:

- 1/4 cup dried hibiscus petals
- 1 cup hot water
- 1 cup frozen mango chunks
- 1 banana
- 1/2 cup orange juice
- 1/2 cup coconut milk
- 1 tablespoon honey or agave syrup (optional, for sweetness)
- Ice cubes

## Instructions:

1. Hibiscus Infusion:
   - Steep hibiscus petals in hot water for 15-20 minutes. Strain to create a vibrant hibiscus infusion.

2. Tropical Tango:
   - In a blender, combine the hibiscus infusion with frozen mango chunks, banana, orange juice, coconut milk, and honey (if using). Blend until the mixture is smooth and dances with tropical flavors.

3. Chill with Ice:
   - Add ice cubes to the blender and blend again until the smoothie reaches a refreshing and chilled consistency.

4. Pour into a Glass:
   - Pour the Mango Tango Hibiscus Smoothie into a glass.

5. Garnish (Optional):
   - Garnish with a hibiscus petal or a slice of mango for a touch of tropical elegance.

6. Sip and Enjoy:
   - Sip and immerse yourself in the tropical tango of mango, hibiscus, and coconut in this vibrant and refreshing smoothie.

# Hibiscus Pomegranate Power Smoothie: A Burst of Antioxidant Richness

The Hibiscus Pomegranate Power Smoothie is a nutritional powerhouse, blending the vibrant hues and antioxidants of hibiscus with the juicy richness of pomegranate. This smoothie is not only a treat for the taste buds but also a refreshing and healthful sip.

## Tips:
1. Pomegranate Prep: Easily extract pomegranate seeds by cutting the fruit in half and tapping the back with a wooden spoon.

2. Greek Yogurt Creaminess: Choose Greek yogurt for added creaminess and a protein boost.

3. Berry Blend Varieties: Experiment with different berry combinations to discover your favorite flavor profile.

4. Natural Sweetness: Taste the smoothie before adding sweeteners, as the natural sugars from the fruits and hibiscus might be sufficient.

## Ingredients:
- 1/4 cup dried hibiscus petals
- 1 cup hot water
- 1/2 cup pomegranate seeds
- 1/2 cup mixed berries (blueberries, raspberries)
- 1 banana
- 1/2 cup Greek yogurt
- 1 tablespoon honey or agave syrup (optional, for sweetness)
- Ice cubes

## Instructions:

1. Hibiscus Infusion:
   - Steep hibiscus petals in hot water for 15-20 minutes. Strain to create a vibrant hibiscus infusion.

2. Antioxidant Fusion:
   - In a blender, combine the hibiscus infusion with pomegranate seeds, mixed berries, banana, Greek yogurt, and honey (if using). Blend until the mixture is smooth and brimming with antioxidant goodness.

3. Chill with Ice:
   - Add ice cubes to the blender and blend again until the smoothie reaches a refreshing and chilled consistency.

4. Pour into a Glass:
   - Pour the Hibiscus Pomegranate Power Smoothie into a glass.

5. Garnish (Optional):
   - Garnish with a hibiscus petal or a sprinkle of pomegranate seeds for an added visual touch.

6. Sip and Enjoy:
   - Sip and revel in the powerful burst of antioxidants and the delightful fusion of hibiscus and pomegranate in this invigorating smoothie.

## Vanilla Hibiscus Protein Smoothie: A Fragrant Protein Boost

The Vanilla Hibiscus Protein Smoothie combines the floral notes of hibiscus with the richness of vanilla and the protein-packed goodness of a protein powder. This smoothie is not only a flavorful delight but also a convenient way to elevate your protein intake.

### Tips:
1. Quality Protein Powder: Choose a high-quality vanilla protein powder to enhance the overall flavor of the smoothie.

2. Almond Milk Creaminess: Opt for almond milk for a creamy texture and a nutty undertone.

3. Natural Sweetness: Taste the smoothie before adding sweeteners, as the natural sugars from the banana and hibiscus might be sufficient.

4. Consistency Control: Adjust the thickness of the smoothie by adding more or fewer ice cubes.

### Ingredients:

- 1/4 cup dried hibiscus petals
- 1 cup hot water
- 1 scoop vanilla protein powder
- 1 banana
- 1/2 cup almond milk
- 1 teaspoon vanilla extract
- 1 tablespoon honey or agave syrup (optional, for sweetness)
- Ice cubes

### Instructions:

1. Hibiscus Infusion:
   - Steep hibiscus petals in hot water for 15-20 minutes. Strain to create a vibrant hibiscus infusion.

2. Protein Powerhouse:
   - In a blender, combine the hibiscus infusion with vanilla protein powder, banana, almond milk, vanilla extract, and honey (if using). Blend until the mixture is smooth and packed with protein goodness.

3. Chill with Ice:
   - Add ice cubes to the blender and blend again until the smoothie reaches a refreshing and chilled consistency.

4. Pour into a Glass:
   - Pour the Vanilla Hibiscus Protein Smoothie into a glass.

5. Garnish (Optional):
   - Garnish with a hibiscus petal or a sprinkle of vanilla protein powder for an added touch.

6. Sip and Enjoy:
   - Sip and relish the fragrant blend of vanilla, hibiscus, and protein in this nourishing and satisfying smoothie.

# Chocolate Hibiscus Delight Smoothie: A Rich and Floral Indulgence

The Chocolate Hibiscus Delight Smoothie is a decadent blend that marries the deep richness of chocolate with the floral elegance of hibiscus. This smoothie is not only a treat for chocolate lovers but also a unique and indulgent experience for anyone seeking a rich and flavorful beverage.

## Tips:

1. Unsweetened Cocoa: Opt for unsweetened cocoa powder to control the sweetness of the smoothie.

2. Almond Milk Creaminess: Almond milk adds a creamy texture and complements the chocolate flavor.

3. Adjusting Sweetness: Taste the smoothie before adding sweeteners, as the natural sugars from the banana and hibiscus might be sufficient.

4. Consistency Control: Customize the thickness of the smoothie by adding more or fewer ice cubes.

## Ingredients:

- 1/4 cup dried hibiscus petals
- 1 cup hot water
- 2 tablespoons unsweetened cocoa powder
- 1 banana
- 1 cup almond milk
- 1 tablespoon honey or agave syrup (optional, for sweetness)
- Ice cubes

## Instructions:

1. Hibiscus Infusion:
   - Steep hibiscus petals in hot water for 15-20 minutes. Strain to create a vibrant hibiscus infusion.

2. Chocolate Infusion:
   - While the hibiscus is steeping, mix cocoa powder with a small amount of hot water to create a smooth chocolate mixture.

3. Blending Magic:
   - In a blender, combine the hibiscus infusion with the cocoa mixture, banana, almond milk, and honey (if using). Blend until the mixture is smooth, rich, and delightfully chocolatey.

4. Chill with Ice:
   - Add ice cubes to the blender and blend again until the smoothie reaches a refreshing and chilled consistency.

5. Pour into a Glass:
   - Pour the Chocolate Hibiscus Delight Smoothie into a glass.

6. Garnish (Optional):
   - Garnish with a hibiscus petal or a sprinkle of cocoa powder for an extra touch of elegance.

7. Sip and Enjoy:
   - Sip and indulge in the luxurious combination of chocolate and hibiscus in this rich and delightful smoothie.

# Hibiscus Spinach Detox Smoothie: A Refreshing Green Cleanse

The Hibiscus Spinach Detox Smoothie is a vibrant green cleanse that combines the detoxifying properties of hibiscus with the nutrient-rich goodness of spinach, cucumber, and apple. This smoothie is not only a refreshing sip but also a nourishing and revitalizing choice for a detox routine.

## Tips:
1. Fresh and Organic: Use fresh, organic produce for maximum nutritional benefits in your detox smoothie.

2. Chia Seed Boost: Chia seeds add a dose of fiber and omega-3 fatty acids; allow them to sit for a few minutes after blending to thicken the smoothie.

3. Lemon Brightness: Adjust the amount of lemon juice based on your preference for tartness.

4. Consistency Control: Customize the thickness of the smoothie by adding more or fewer ice cubes.

## Ingredients:
- 1/4 cup dried hibiscus petals
- 1 cup hot water
- Handful of fresh spinach leaves
- 1/2 cucumber, peeled and sliced
- 1/2 green apple, cored and sliced
- Juice of 1 lemon
- 1 tablespoon chia seeds
- Ice cubes

## Instructions:

1. Hibiscus Infusion:
   - Steep hibiscus petals in hot water for 15-20 minutes. Strain to create a vibrant hibiscus infusion.

2. Green Cleanse:
   - In a blender, combine the hibiscus infusion with fresh spinach leaves, cucumber slices, green apple slices, lemon juice, and chia seeds. Blend until the mixture is smooth and packed with detoxifying goodness.

3. Chill with Ice:
   - Add ice cubes to the blender and blend again until the smoothie reaches a refreshing and chilled consistency.

4. Pour into a Glass:
   - Pour the Hibiscus Spinach Detox Smoothie into a glass.

5. Garnish (Optional):
   - Garnish with a hibiscus petal or a slice of cucumber for a touch of freshness.

6. Sip and Enjoy:
   - Sip and relish the refreshing and detoxifying blend of hibiscus, spinach, and green goodness in this revitalizing smoothie.

# Coconut Berry Hibiscus Smoothie: A Tropical Berry Bliss

The Coconut Berry Hibiscus Smoothie is a tropical paradise in a glass, combining the floral notes of hibiscus with the lusciousness of mixed berries and the creaminess of coconut. This smoothie is not only a treat for the taste buds but also a mini vacation to a tropical oasis.

## Tips:
1. Coconut Milk Creaminess: Opt for full-fat coconut milk for a richer and creamier texture.

2. Shredded Coconut Crunch: Shredded coconut adds a delightful crunch; toast it for extra flavor.

3. Natural Sweetness: Taste the smoothie before adding sweeteners, as the natural sugars from the berries and hibiscus might be sufficient.

4. Consistency Control: Customize the thickness of the smoothie by adding more or fewer ice cubes.

## Ingredients:

- 1/4 cup dried hibiscus petals
- 1 cup hot water
- 1/2 cup mixed berries (strawberries, blueberries, raspberries)
- 1/2 cup coconut milk
- 1 banana
- 1 tablespoon shredded coconut (optional)
- 1 tablespoon honey or agave syrup (optional, for sweetness)
- Ice cubes

## Instructions:

1. Hibiscus Infusion:
   - Steep hibiscus petals in hot water for 15-20 minutes. Strain to create a vibrant hibiscus infusion.

2. Tropical Berry Blend:
   - In a blender, combine the hibiscus infusion with mixed berries, coconut milk, banana, shredded coconut (if using), and honey (if using). Blend until the mixture is smooth, tropical, and bursting with berry goodness.

3. Chill with Ice:
   - Add ice cubes to the blender and blend again until the smoothie reaches a refreshing and chilled consistency.

4. Pour into a Glass:
   - Pour the Coconut Berry Hibiscus Smoothie into a glass.

5. Garnish (Optional):
   - Garnish with a hibiscus petal or a sprinkle of shredded coconut for a tropical touch.

6. Sip and Enjoy:
   - Sip and indulge in the tropical berry bliss of this Coconut Berry Hibiscus Smoothie.

# Hibiscus Matcha Fusion Smoothie with a Surprise Twist

The Hibiscus Matcha Fusion Smoothie is a surprising and exotic blend that combines the floral notes of hibiscus with the earthiness of matcha and a hint of cayenne for a kick. This smoothie is not only a treat for the adventurous palate but also a flavorful journey with every sip.

## Tips:
1. Quality Matcha: Choose high-quality matcha powder for a more vibrant and authentic flavor.

2. Cayenne Kick: Adjust the amount of cayenne pepper based on your spice tolerance for a delightful surprise.

3. Pineapple Sweetness: The pineapple chunks add natural sweetness; taste before adding sweeteners.

4. Consistency Control: Customize the thickness of the smoothie by adding more or fewer ice cubes.

## Ingredients:
- 1/4 cup dried hibiscus petals
- 1 cup hot water
- 1 teaspoon matcha powder
- 1/2 cup pineapple chunks (fresh or frozen)
- 1 banana
- 1/2 cup coconut milk
- 1 tablespoon honey or agave syrup (optional, for sweetness)
- A pinch of cayenne pepper (surprise ingredient)
- Ice cubes

## Instructions:

1. Hibiscus Infusion:
   - Steep hibiscus petals in hot water for 15-20 minutes. Strain to create a vibrant hibiscus infusion.

2. Matcha Marvel:
   - While the hibiscus is steeping, whisk matcha powder in a small amount of hot water to create a smooth matcha mixture.

3. Fusion Magic:
   - In a blender, combine the hibiscus infusion with the matcha mixture, pineapple chunks, banana, coconut milk, honey (if using), and a surprising pinch of cayenne pepper. Blend until the mixture is smooth, exotic, and tantalizing to the taste buds.

4. Chill with Ice:
   - Add ice cubes to the blender and blend again until the smoothie reaches a refreshing and chilled consistency.

5. Pour into a Glass:
   - Pour the Hibiscus Matcha Fusion Smoothie into a glass.

6. Garnish (Optional):
   - Garnish with a hibiscus petal or a sprinkle of matcha powder for an extra element of surprise.

# The Cherry Almond Hibiscus Smoothie: A Nutty Berry Symphony

The Cherry Almond Hibiscus Smoothie is a nutty and fruity symphony that combines the tartness of cherries with the richness of almonds and the floral notes of hibiscus. This smoothie is not only a treat for the taste buds but also a nutritious and satisfying choice for any time of the day.

## Tips:
1. Soaked Almonds: Soak almonds in water overnight or for a few hours for a creamier texture and enhanced nutrient absorption.

2. Cherry Goodness: Adjust the quantity of cherries based on your preference for sweetness and tartness.

3. Almond Milk Creaminess: Opt for unsweetened almond milk for better control over the sweetness of the smoothie.

4. Natural Sweetness: Taste the smoothie before adding sweeteners, as the natural sugars from the cherries and hibiscus might be sufficient.

5. Consistency Control: Customize the thickness of the smoothie by adding more or fewer ice cubes.

## Ingredients:

- 1/4 cup dried hibiscus petals
- 1 cup hot water
- 1/2 cup frozen cherries
- 1 banana
- 1/4 cup almonds, soaked
- 1/2 cup almond milk
- 1 tablespoon honey or agave syrup (optional, for sweetness)
- Ice cubes

## Instructions:

1. Hibiscus Infusion:
   - Steep hibiscus petals in hot water for 15-20 minutes. Strain to create a vibrant hibiscus infusion.

2. Cherry Almond Symphony:
   - In a blender, combine the hibiscus infusion with frozen cherries, banana, soaked almonds, almond milk, and honey (if using). Blend until the mixture is smooth, nutty, and brimming with cherry goodness.

3. Chill with Ice:
   - Add ice cubes to the blender and blend again until the smoothie reaches a refreshing and chilled consistency.

4. Pour into a Glass:
   - Pour the Cherry Almond Hibiscus Smoothie into a glass.

5. Garnish (Optional):
   - Garnish with a hibiscus petal or a few whole cherries for an elegant touch.

6. Sip and Enjoy:
   - Sip and relish the harmonious blend of cherries, almonds, and hibiscus in this delightful and nutty smoothie.

## Savory Hibiscus Tomato Basil Smoothie

The "Hibiscus Tomato Basil Fusion Smoothie" – a daring blend that harmonizes robust hibiscus tea with fresh tomatoes, basil, and savory accents. This unexpectedly refreshing concoction invites you to explore a symphony of flavors, balancing floral sweetness with the earthy richness of tomatoes and basil. Perfectly chilled and garnished for visual flair, it's a unique smoothie experience that defies expectations.

### Tips:

1. Bold Hibiscus Tea:
   - Choose a robust hibiscus tea for a more intense floral flavor.
2. Fresh is Best:
   - Use fresh tomatoes, basil, cucumber, and red onion for vibrant taste.
3. Balance Savory and Sweet:
   - Adjust ingredient quantities to find the right savory-sweet ratio.
4. Chill for Refreshment:
   - Refrigerate ingredients for a colder, more refreshing experience.
5. Texture Play:
   - Experiment with ice or hibiscus tea amounts for desired thickness.
6. Creative Garnish:
   - Elevate presentation with basil leaves or cucumber slices.

### Variations:

1. Spicy Kick:
   - Add red pepper flakes or hot sauce for heat.
2. Creamy Twist:
   - Blend in Greek yogurt or avocado for richness.
3. Protein Boost:
   - Include plant-based protein powder.

### Ingredients:

- 1 cup brewed and cooled hibiscus tea
- 1 cup tomato juice
- Handful of fresh basil leaves
- 1/2 cucumber, peeled and diced
- 1/2 small red onion, diced
- 1 clove garlic, minced
- 1 tablespoon olive oil
- Salt and pepper to taste
- Ice cubes (optional)

### Instructions:

1. Brew hibiscus tea and allow it to cool.

2. In a blender, combine the cooled hibiscus tea, tomato juice, basil leaves, diced cucumber, diced red onion, minced garlic, and olive oil.

3. Blend until smooth. If the mixture is too thick, you can add a bit of water or more hibiscus tea to reach your desired consistency.

4. Season with salt and pepper to taste. If you prefer a colder drink, you can add ice cubes and blend again until smooth.

5. Pour into a glass and garnish with a fresh basil leaf for an extra touch.

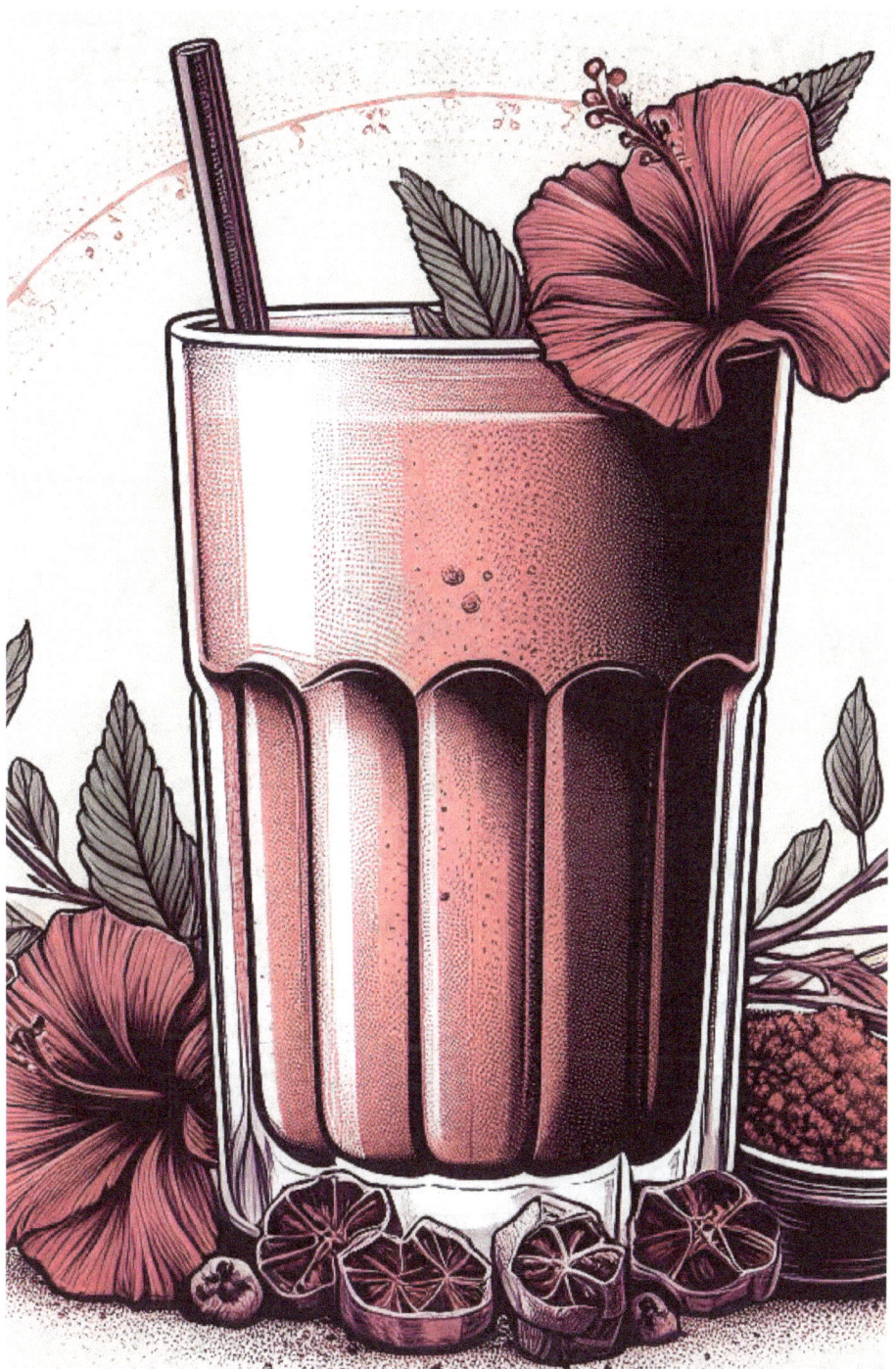

# Mocktails & Cocktails

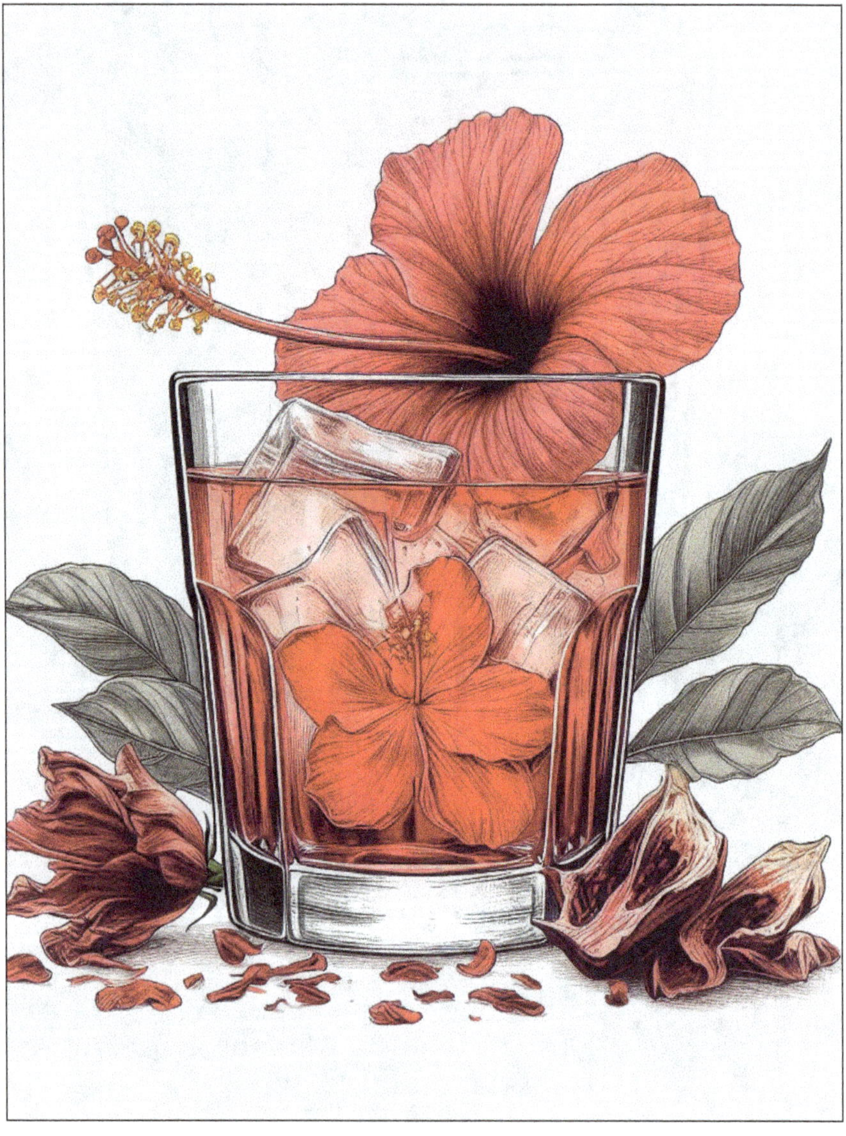

# Hibiscus Sparkler: A Refreshing Floral Fizz

The Hibiscus Sparkler is a refreshing and bubbly drink that combines the floral notes of hibiscus tea with the effervescence of sparkling water. A splash of lemon juice adds a zesty twist, while fresh mint leaves contribute a burst of coolness. This sparkler is not only a delightful beverage but also a perfect companion for warm, sunny days.

## Tips:
1. Brew Strong Hibiscus Tea: For a more pronounced hibiscus flavor, brew the tea a bit stronger than usual.

2. Adjust Lemon Splash: Customize the amount of lemon juice based on your preference for acidity.

3. Minty Freshness: Crush the mint leaves slightly before adding to release their aromatic oils.

4. Experiment with Sparkling Water: Try different types of sparkling water, such as plain, citrus-flavored, or berry-infused, to find your favorite combination.

## Ingredients:

- Hibiscus tea (cooled)
- Sparkling water
- Splash of lemon juice
- Fresh mint leaves
- Ice cubes

## Instructions:

1. Prepare Hibiscus Tea:
   - Brew hibiscus tea and let it cool to room temperature or refrigerate for a chilled base.

2. Mix and Sparkle:
   - In a glass, combine hibiscus tea with sparkling water. Add a splash of lemon juice for a citrusy kick.

3. Garnish with Mint:
   - Drop in a few fresh mint leaves for a burst of freshness.

4. Chill with Ice:
   - Add ice cubes to the glass to keep the sparkler cool.

5. Stir Gently:
   - Give it a gentle stir to mix the flavors.

6. Sip and Enjoy:
   - Sip and relish the effervescent and floral delight of the Hibiscus Sparkler.

## Tropical Hibiscus Cooler: A Sip of Exotic Paradise

Indulge in the blissful escape of our Tropical Hibiscus Cooler – a tantalizing blend of chilled hibiscus tea, pineapple, and orange juices. This refreshing elixir, with a hint of optional passion fruit, invites you to savor the tropical symphony of flavors. As you sip over ice, fresh mint leaves dance through each drop, creating a cool breeze of exotic delight. Garnished with a sprig of mint, this beverage transforms any moment into a brief escape to a sun-kissed oasis. Cheers to the Tropical Hibiscus Cooler – your passport to a sip of paradise.

### Ingredients:

- Hibiscus tea (cooled)
- Pineapple juice
- Orange juice
- Passion fruit juice (optional)
- Ice cubes
- Fresh mint leaves for garnish

### Instructions

1. Mix equal parts hibiscus tea, pineapple juice, and orange juice in a pitcher.

2. Optionally, add a splash of passion fruit juice for extra tropical flavor.

3. Pour the Tropical Hibiscus Cooler over ice in glasses.

4. Garnish with fresh mint leaves for a burst of freshness.

5. Stir gently and enjoy your tropical paradise in a glass.

### Variations

**1. Coconut Bliss Tropical Hibiscus Cooler:**
- Combine the Tropical Hibiscus Cooler with coconut water or coconut milk for a creamy and exotic twist. Garnish with shredded coconut for an added touch of tropical bliss.

**2. Mango Tango Tropical Hibiscus Cooler:**
- Introduce the sweet and luscious flavor of mango by adding mango puree or mango chunks to the Tropical Hibiscus Cooler. This variation enhances the tropical experience with a burst of fruity goodness.

**3. Pineapple Ginger Tropical Hibiscus Refresher:**
- Infuse the Tropical Hibiscus Cooler with the zing of freshly grated ginger and the tropical sweetness of pineapple juice. This variation adds a spicy and fruity kick to your cooler, creating a well-balanced and invigorating drink.

## Passionfruit Hibiscus Fizz: Tropical Symphony in a Glass

Immerse yourself in the tropical allure of our Passionfruit Hibiscus Fizz, where the vibrant notes of passionfruit and the delicate elegance of hibiscus converge in a harmonious dance. This effervescent elixir, crowned with the light sparkle of soda water and a hint of agave syrup, offers a refreshing escape to a sun-kissed paradise with every sip. The deep crimson hue and the sweet-tart melody create a sensory journey, making this fizz a celebration of tropical elegance.

### Ingredients:

- 1 cup hibiscus tea (cooled)
- 1/2 cup passionfruit juice
- 1/2 cup soda water
- 1-2 tablespoons agave syrup (adjust to taste)
- Ice cubes
- Passionfruit wedge or hibiscus petal for garnish (optional)

### Instructions:

1. Brew Hibiscus Tea:
   - Brew a cup of hibiscus tea and let it cool to room temperature. You can use hibiscus tea bags or dried hibiscus petals.

2. Prepare Passionfruit Juice:
   - Extract the juice from fresh passionfruit or use store-bought passionfruit juice.

3. Combine Ingredients:
   - In a glass, combine the cooled hibiscus tea with passionfruit juice. Stir well to mix the flavors.

4. Add Soda Water:
   - Pour in the soda water to add a delightful fizziness to the drink.

5. Sweeten with Agave Syrup:
   - Add agave syrup to sweeten the fizz. Start with one tablespoon and adjust according to your preferred level of sweetness.

6. Mix Well:
   - Stir the ingredients well to ensure the agave syrup is fully incorporated.

7. Chill with Ice:
   - Add ice cubes to the glass to keep the Passionfruit Hibiscus Fizz cool.

8. Garnish (Optional):
   - Garnish with a wedge of fresh passionfruit or a hibiscus petal for a decorative touch.

9. Sip and Enjoy:
   - Sip and revel in the tropical elegance of the Passionfruit Hibiscus Fizz. Cheers to a burst of exotic refreshment!

### Variations:

1. Minty Fresh Twist:
   - Muddle a few fresh mint leaves in the glass before adding the ingredients. The herbal essence of mint complements the tropical flavors, adding a layer of cool freshness.

2. Ginger Spice Infusion:
   - Infuse the hibiscus tea with a slice of fresh ginger for a subtle spice. This variation adds a warm kick, balancing the sweetness of passionfruit.

3. - Replace the soda water with coconut water for a more tropical and hydrating experience. Garnish with shredded coconut for added texture.

## Mango Hibiscus Splash: A Tropical Tango of Flavors

Indulge in the vibrant allure of our Mango Hibiscus Splash – a tantalizing fusion of fresh mango puree, hibiscus infusion, and a zesty squeeze of lime. This refreshing elixir is a dance of tropical sweetness and floral sophistication, inviting you to savor the essence of a sun-soaked paradise with every sip.

In the Mango Hibiscus Splash, the lusciousness of ripe mangoes intertwines with the deep crimson hues and subtle tartness of hibiscus, creating a symphony of flavors that plays delicately on your palate. The addition of a lime squeeze adds a burst of citrusy brightness, elevating the overall experience to a tropical tango.

Served over ice and garnished with a slice of lime or a hibiscus petal, this Mango Hibiscus Splash is not merely a beverage; it's an escape. Each sip transports you to a world where the air is filled with the fragrance of blooming flowers and the sun kisses your skin.

Perfect for a leisurely afternoon by the pool or as a lively companion to social gatherings, the Mango Hibiscus Splash is a celebration of tropical indulgence. Cheers to the artistry of flavors and the joy of sipping a tropical tango in a glass – a refreshing splash awaits.

---

### Ingredients:

- 1 cup fresh mango puree
- 1 cup hibiscus tea infusion (cooled)
- Juice of 1 lime
- Ice cubes
- Hibiscus petal or lime slice for garnish (optional)

### Instructions:

1. Prepare Hibiscus Tea Infusion:
   - Brew a cup of hibiscus tea and let it cool to room temperature or refrigerate for a chilled infusion.

2. Extract Mango Puree:
   - Peel and dice fresh mangoes, then blend to a smooth puree.

3. Combine Ingredients:
   - In a pitcher or glass, mix the fresh mango puree with the cooled hibiscus tea infusion.

4. Squeeze Lime:
   - Add the juice of one lime to the mixture. Adjust the lime juice according to your preferred level of tartness.

5. Stir Well:
   - Stir the ingredients well to ensure a harmonious blend of mango, hibiscus, and lime.

6. Chill with Ice:
   - Add ice cubes to the glass or pitcher to keep the Mango Hibiscus Splash refreshingly cool.

7. Garnish (Optional):
   - Garnish with a hibiscus petal or a slice of lime for a decorative touch.

8. Sip and Enjoy:
   - Savor the tropical tango of flavors with each delightful sip of the Mango Hibiscus Splash.

---

### Variation.

1. Basil Mango Bliss:
   - Muddle a few fresh basil leaves in the glass before adding the ingredients. Basil adds a subtle herbal note that complements the tropical flavors.

# Berry Hibiscus Crush: A Symphony of Berries and Blooms

Embark on a journey of vibrant flavors with our Berry Hibiscus Crush – a refreshing blend of mixed berry puree, hibiscus tea, crushed ice, and a citrusy twist of orange. This invigorating elixir is a symphony of sweet berries, floral hibiscus, and zesty orange, creating a crush-worthy beverage that captivates the senses.

## Ingredients:

- 1 cup mixed berry puree (strawberries, blueberries, raspberries)
- 1 cup hibiscus tea (cooled)
- Crushed ice
- Twist of orange peel for garnish
- Fresh berries for garnish (optional)

## Instructions:

1. Prepare Mixed Berry Puree:
   - Blend a combination of strawberries, blueberries, and raspberries to create a smooth mixed berry puree.

2. Brew Hibiscus Tea:
   - Brew a cup of hibiscus tea and let it cool to room temperature.

3. Combine Ingredients:
   - In a glass or pitcher, mix the mixed berry puree with the cooled hibiscus tea.

4. Crush Ice:
   - Add crushed ice to the glass or pitcher, filling it generously to create a refreshing, chilled base.

5. Stir Well:
   - Stir the ingredients well to ensure the berry puree and hibiscus tea are thoroughly combined.

6. Garnish:
   - Twist a strip of orange peel over the drink to release its citrus oils. Drop the peel into the crush for added aroma.
   - Optionally, garnish with fresh berries for a burst of color.

7. Serve and Enjoy:
   - Sip and relish the Berry Hibiscus Crush, a delightful fusion of berries, hibiscus, and citrus.

## Variations.

1. Minty Berry Burst:
   - Muddle a few fresh mint leaves in the glass before adding the ingredients. Mint adds a refreshing herbal note to the crush.

2. Gingerberry Infusion:
   - Infuse the hibiscus tea with a slice of fresh ginger for a hint of warmth. This variation introduces a subtle spicy kick.

3. Coconut Berry Bliss:
   - Replace regular crushed ice with coconut water ice cubes for a tropical twist. Garnish with shredded coconut for added texture.

4. Basil Berry Crush:
   - Add a few basil leaves to the berry puree for a herbal undertone that complements the sweetness of the berries.

Feel free to experiment with these variations or create your own unique twists on the Berry Hibiscus Crush. Whether enjoyed on a sunny afternoon or shared at gatherings, this crush is a celebration of fruity delights and floral blooms. Cheers to the art of crafting refreshing beverages!

# Cucumber Hibiscus Refresher: A Symphony of Cool Elegance

Dive into a world of cool sophistication with our Cucumber Hibiscus Refresher – a harmonious blend of crisp cucumber slices, hibiscus water, delicate elderflower syrup, and a splash of effervescent tonic. This invigorating elixir is a celebration of botanical freshness and floral notes, creating a refresher that elegantly dances on the palate.

## Ingredients:

- Cucumber slices
- Hibiscus water (hibiscus tea cooled to room temperature)
- Elderflower syrup
- Splash of tonic water
- Ice cubes
- Fresh mint leaves for garnish

## Instructions:

1. Prepare Hibiscus Water:
   - Brew a cup of hibiscus tea and let it cool to room temperature or refrigerate for a chilled infusion.

2. Slice Cucumbers:
   - Thinly slice fresh cucumbers to release their crisp and refreshing essence.

3. Combine Ingredients:
   - In a glass, combine cucumber slices, hibiscus water, and a drizzle of elderflower syrup.

4. Add Tonic Water:
   - Pour a splash of tonic water over the cucumber and hibiscus mix to add a light effervescence.

5. Stir Gently:
   - Stir the ingredients gently to blend the flavors while maintaining the crisp texture of the cucumber.

6. Chill with Ice:
   - Add ice cubes to the glass to keep the Cucumber Hibiscus Refresher refreshingly cool.

7. Garnish with Mint:
   - Garnish with fresh mint leaves for a burst of herbal aroma and visual appeal.

8. Sip and Enjoy:
   - Savor the cool elegance of the Cucumber Hibiscus Refresher – a perfect sip for moments of relaxation.

## Variations:

1. Gingered Cucumber Bloom:
   - Infuse the hibiscus water with a hint of fresh ginger for a subtle warmth that complements the coolness of cucumber.

2. Citrus Cucumber Spark:
   - Squeeze a wedge of lime or add a few citrus slices for a zesty twist that brightens the overall flavor profile.

3. Minted Elderflower Breeze:
   - Muddle a few fresh mint leaves in the glass before adding the ingredients. This variation enhances the herbal notes of elderflower.

4. Basil Cucumber Symphony:
   - Add a few basil leaves to the mix for a herbal undertone that adds depth to the refresher.

# Coconut Hibiscus Elixir: A Tropical Symphony in a Glass

Immerse yourself in the exotic allure of our Coconut Hibiscus Elixir – a divine fusion of pure coconut water, hibiscus syrup, the zesty embrace of lime juice, and a hint of invigorating ginger. This enchanting elixir is a celebration of tropical indulgence, crafting a symphony of flavors that dance gracefully on your palate.

## Ingredients:

- Coconut water
- Hibiscus syrup
- Lime juice
- Dash of ginger (freshly grated or ginger syrup)
- Ice cubes
- Hibiscus petal or lime wedge for garnish

## Instructions:

1. Prepare Hibiscus Syrup:
   - Create hibiscus syrup by combining hibiscus tea with an equal amount of sugar, simmering until dissolved, and letting it cool.

2. Combine Ingredients:
   - In a glass, mix coconut water with a drizzle of hibiscus syrup.

3. Add Lime Juice:
   - Squeeze fresh lime juice into the mix, adjusting to your desired level of tartness.

4. Dash of Ginger:
   - Add a dash of freshly grated ginger or ginger syrup to infuse a subtle warmth and spice.

5. Stir Well:
   - Stir the ingredients well to ensure a harmonious blend of coconut, hibiscus, lime, and ginger.

6. Chill with Ice:
   - Add ice cubes to the glass, creating a refreshing base for the Coconut Hibiscus Elixir.

7. Garnish:
   - Garnish with a hibiscus petal or a wedge of lime for a touch of visual elegance.

8. Sip and Enjoy:
   - Indulge in the tropical symphony of the Coconut Hibiscus Elixir, a sip of paradise in every glass.

## Variations:.

1. Minty Coconut Breeze:
   - Muddle a few fresh mint leaves in the glass before adding the ingredients. Mint adds a refreshing herbal note.

2. Pineapple Hibiscus Fusion:
   - Include a splash of pineapple juice for a sweet and tangy twist that complements the coconut and hibiscus.

3. Vanilla Hibiscus Dream:
   - Add a drop of vanilla extract for a subtle sweetness that enhances the overall tropical experience.

4. Chili Lime Coconut Kick:
   - Infuse the elixir with a tiny pinch of chili powder or a slice of fresh chili for a spicy kick balanced by the citrusy lime.

# Blueberry Basil Hibiscus Bliss: A Symphony of Berry and Herb Elegance

Embark on a journey of exquisite flavors with our Blueberry Basil Hibiscus Bliss – a divine blend of luscious blueberry juice, hibiscus tea, the aromatic essence of fresh basil, and a delicate touch of honey. This enchanting elixir is a celebration of berry sweetness and herbal sophistication, creating a blissful experience that dances gracefully on your palate.

## Ingredients:

- Blueberry juice
- Hibiscus tea (cooled)
- Fresh basil leaves
- Touch of honey (adjust to taste)
- Ice cubes
- Fresh blueberries and basil sprig for garnish

## Instructions:

1. Brew Hibiscus Tea:
   - Brew a cup of hibiscus tea and let it cool to room temperature or refrigerate for a chilled infusion.

2. Prepare Blueberry Juice:
   - Extract fresh blueberry juice by blending blueberries and straining the mixture to get a smooth juice.

3. Muddle Basil:
   - In a glass, muddle a few fresh basil leaves to release their aromatic oils.

4. Combine Ingredients:
   - Pour blueberry juice and cooled hibiscus tea into the glass with muddled basil.

5. Add Honey:
   - Add a touch of honey to sweeten the blend. Adjust the amount based on your preferred level of sweetness.

6. Stir Well:
   - Stir the ingredients well to infuse the flavors of blueberry, hibiscus, basil, and honey.

7. Chill with Ice:
   - Add ice cubes to the glass for a refreshing and chilled Blueberry Basil Hibiscus Bliss.

8. Garnish:
   - Garnish with fresh blueberries and a sprig of basil for a burst of visual appeal.

9. Sip and Enjoy:
   - Delight in the symphony of flavors with each sip of the Blueberry Basil Hibiscus Bliss – a heavenly combination of berries and herbs.

## Variations:

1. Citrusy Basil Burst:
   - Squeeze a wedge of lime or add a splash of orange juice for a citrusy twist that complements the blueberries and basil.

2. Minty Blueberry Infusion:
   - Replace or combine basil with fresh mint leaves for an additional layer of herbal freshness.

3. Vanilla Berry Serenity:
   - Add a drop of vanilla extract for a subtle sweetness that enhances the overall berry experience.

4. Ginger Blueberry Zing:
   - Infuse the elixir with a dash of freshly grated ginger for a hint of spice that harmonizes with the sweet blueberries.

# Ginger Lemongrass Hibiscus Infusion: A Zesty and Floral Elixir

Indulge in the invigorating fusion of flavors with our Ginger Lemongrass Hibiscus Infusion – a vibrant blend of spicy ginger, citrusy lemongrass, and the deep, floral notes of hibiscus. This aromatic elixir promises a refreshing experience that awakens the senses and soothes the soul.

## Ingredients:

- 1 tablespoon dried hibiscus petals or hibiscus tea bag
- 1 tablespoon fresh lemongrass, chopped
- 1 teaspoon fresh ginger, grated
- Honey or agave syrup (optional, to taste)
- Hot water
- Lemon wedge for garnish

## Instructions:

1. Prepare Hibiscus Tea Base:
   - If using dried hibiscus petals, place them in a teapot or infuser. Pour hot water over the hibiscus and let it steep for 5-7 minutes. If using a hibiscus tea bag, steep it in hot water for the recommended time.

2. Add Lemongrass and Ginger:
   - Add the chopped lemongrass and grated ginger to the hibiscus tea base. Allow the flavors to infuse for an additional 3-5 minutes.

3. Strain or Remove Tea Bag:
   - Strain the infusion to remove hibiscus petals, lemongrass, and ginger, or remove the tea bag, depending on your preparation.

4. Sweeten (Optional):
   - Sweeten the infusion with honey or agave syrup if desired. Adjust the sweetness to your preference.

5. Garnish:
   - Garnish with a fresh lemon wedge for an extra burst of citrus aroma.

6. Serve and Sip:
   - Pour the Ginger Lemongrass Hibiscus Infusion into your favorite teacup and savor the zesty, floral medley.

## Variations:

1. Chilled Delight:
   - After steeping, let the infusion cool and refrigerate it for a refreshing iced version.

2. Minty Twist:
   - Add a few fresh mint leaves to the infusion for a cooling and herbal note.

3. Orange Blossom Elegance:
   - Include a twist of orange peel during steeping for a subtle citrusy addition.

4. Cayenne Kick:
   - For an adventurous touch, add a pinch of cayenne pepper to spice up the infusion.

## Pomegranate Hibiscus Breeze: A Refreshing Symphony of Fruity Elegance

Savor the delightful harmony of flavors with our Pomegranate Hibiscus Breeze – a rejuvenating blend of rich pomegranate juice, the deep floral notes of hibiscus infusion, effervescent sparkling water, and a zesty twist of lemon. This enchanting elixir promises a cooling breeze of fruity elegance that captivates the senses.

### Ingredients:

- 1/2 cup pomegranate juice
- 1/2 cup hibiscus infusion (cooled)
- 1/2 cup sparkling water
- Twist of lemon peel
- Ice cubes
- Pomegranate arils for garnish (optional)

### Instructions:

1. Prepare Hibiscus Infusion:
   - Brew a cup of hibiscus tea and let it cool to room temperature or refrigerate for a chilled infusion.

2. Combine Ingredients:
   - In a glass, mix pomegranate juice and cooled hibiscus infusion.

3. Add Sparkling Water:
   - Pour sparkling water into the mix to introduce a lively effervescence.

4. Twist of Lemon:
   - Add a twist of lemon peel to enhance the citrusy aroma. Ensure it is a thin strip of peel, avoiding the bitter white pith.

5. Chill with Ice:
   - Drop ice cubes into the glass to keep the Pomegranate Hibiscus Breeze cool and refreshing.

6. Garnish (Optional):
   - Optionally, garnish with pomegranate arils for a burst of color and added texture.

7. Stir Gently:
   - Stir the ingredients gently to combine the fruity, floral, and effervescent elements.

8. Sip and Enjoy:
   - Savor the symphony of fruity elegance with each sip of the Pomegranate Hibiscus Breeze – a cool and refreshing indulgence.

### Variations:

1. **Minty Pomegranate Burst:**
   - Muddle a few fresh mint leaves in the glass before adding the ingredients. Mint adds a refreshing herbal note.

2. **Gingered Hibiscus Delight:**
   - Infuse the hibiscus tea with a hint of freshly grated ginger for a subtle warmth.

3. **Berry Bliss Infusion:**
   - Enhance the hibiscus infusion with a handful of mixed berries for an extra layer of fruity goodness.

4. **Vanilla Pomegranate Serenity:**
   - Add a drop of vanilla extract for a touch of sweetness that complements the pomegranate.

Feel free to explore these variations or create your own to tailor the Pomegranate Hibiscus Breeze to your taste preferences. Whether enjoyed on a warm afternoon or as a vibrant addition to gatherings, this refreshing breeze promises a symphony of delightful flavors. Cheers to the art of crafting invigorating beverages!

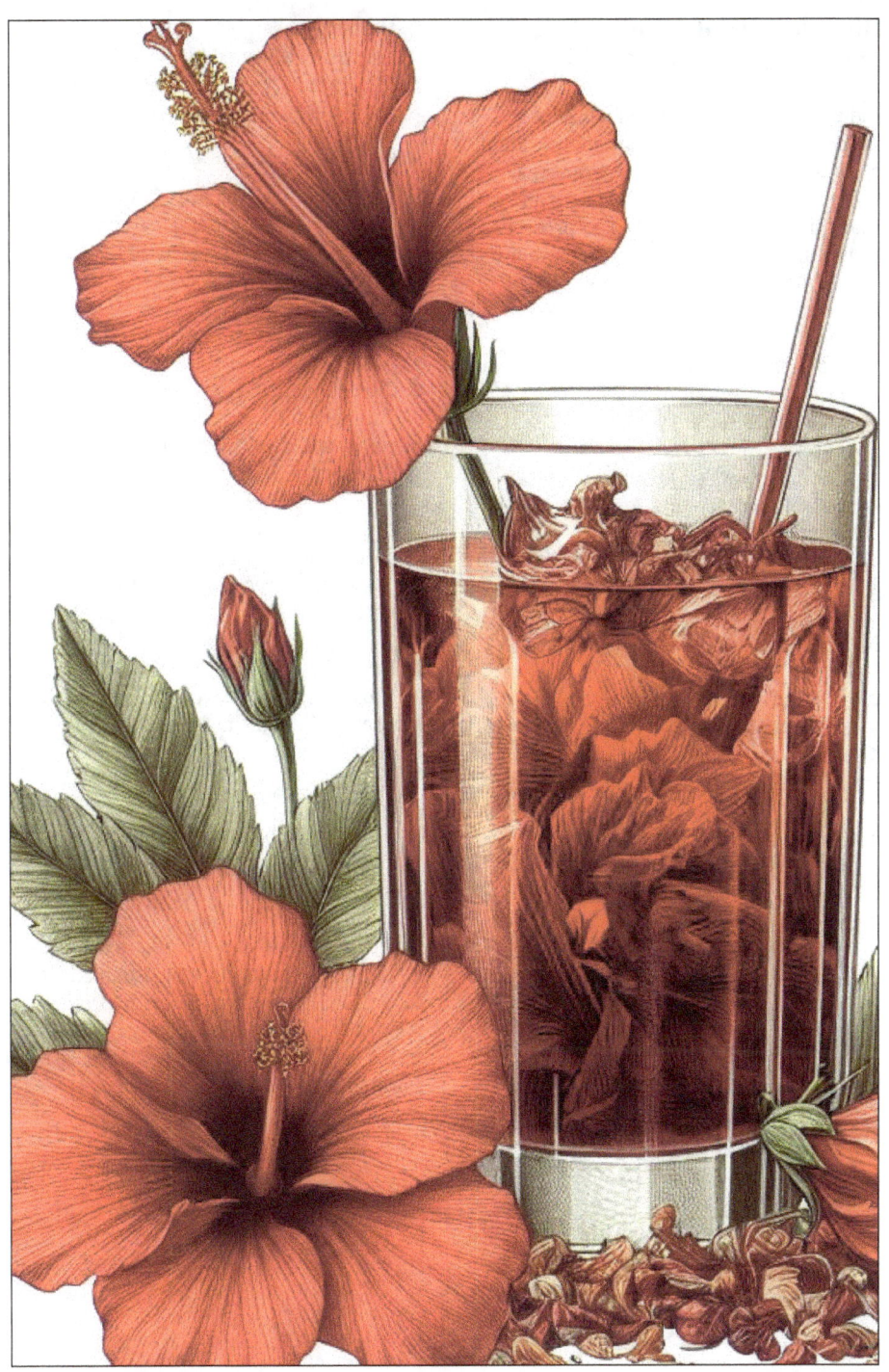

# Hibiscus Rose Martini: A Floral Symphony in a Glass

Indulge in the sophisticated allure of the Hibiscus Rose Martini, a captivating blend of hibiscus-infused vodka, fragrant rose water, delicate elderflower liqueur, and a sparkling finish with a splash of prosecco. This crafted martini is a floral symphony that invites you to savor the elegance of botanical flavors.

## Ingredients:

- 2 oz hibiscus-infused vodka
- 1/2 oz rose water
- 1/2 oz elderflower liqueur
- Splash of prosecco
- Ice cubes
- Edible flower (such as a rose petal) for garnish

## Instructions:

1. Prepare Hibiscus-Infused Vodka:
   - Infuse vodka with dried hibiscus petals. Allow it to steep for at least 24 hours, then strain to obtain hibiscus-infused vodka.

2. Combine Ingredients:
   - In a mixing glass, combine hibiscus-infused vodka, rose water, and elderflower liqueur.

3. Shake Well:
   - Shake the mixture vigorously with ice to chill and blend the floral flavors.

4. Strain into Martini Glass:
   - Strain the martini into a chilled martini glass.

5. Top with Prosecco:
   - Finish the martini with a gentle splash of prosecco for a touch of effervescence.

6. Garnish Elegantly:
   - Garnish with an edible flower, such as a delicate rose petal, for an elegant visual touch.

7. Sip and Enjoy:
   - Savor the Hibiscus Rose Martini, a refined libation that marries the floral notes of hibiscus and rose with the subtle sweetness of elderflower.

## Variations:

1. **Citrus Bloom Twist:**
   - Enhance the martini with a hint of citrus by adding a twist of grapefruit or orange peel.

2. **Thyme-Infused Elegance:**
   - Infuse the hibiscus-infused vodka with a sprig of fresh thyme for an herbal undertone.

3. **Lavender Whisper:**
   - Float a few dried lavender buds on the surface of the martini for a whisper of lavender aroma.

4. **Gingered Petal Passion:**
   - Add a touch of ginger syrup for a subtle warmth that complements the floral profile.

Whether enjoyed as a prelude to an evening or a centerpiece at a sophisticated affair, the Hibiscus Rose Martini promises a journey of refined indulgence. Cheers to the art of mixology and the pleasure of floral-infused libations!

## Passion Hibiscus Margarita: A Tropical Fiesta in a Glass

Transport your taste buds to a sun-soaked paradise with the Passion Hibiscus Margarita, a vibrant concoction featuring the allure of hibiscus-infused tequila, the exotic sweetness of passionfruit puree, the citrusy kick of triple sec, and a splash of zesty lime juice. This tropical margarita is a celebration of flavors that invites you to savor the fiesta in every sip.

### Ingredients:

- 2 oz hibiscus-infused tequila
- 1 oz passionfruit puree
- 3/4 oz triple sec
- 3/4 oz fresh lime juice
- Agave syrup (optional, for sweetness)
- Ice cubes
- Salt or Tajín for rimming (optional)
- Lime wheel and hibiscus petal for garnish

### Instructions:

1. Prepare Hibiscus-Infused Tequila:
   - Infuse tequila with dried hibiscus petals. Allow it to steep for at least 24 hours, then strain to obtain hibiscus-infused tequila.

2. Rim the Glass (Optional):
   - If desired, rim a glass with salt or Tajín by moistening the rim with a lime wedge and dipping it into the seasoning.

3. Combine Ingredients:
   - In a shaker, combine hibiscus-infused tequila, passionfruit puree, triple sec, and fresh lime juice.

4. Add Agave Syrup (Optional):
   - Depending on your sweetness preference, add agave syrup to the shaker. Shake well to combine.

5. Shake Vigorously:
   - Shake the mixture with ice vigorously to chill and meld the flavors.

6. Strain into Glass:
   - Strain the margarita into the prepared glass filled with ice.

7. Garnish Creatively:
   - Garnish with a lime wheel and a hibiscus petal for a visually striking presentation.

8. Sip and Revel:
   - Immerse yourself in the tropical fiesta with every sip of the Passion Hibiscus Margarita, a harmonious blend of floral, fruity, and citrusy notes.

### Variations:

**1. Spicy Hibiscus Kick:**
   - Add a slice of jalapeño to the shaker for a spicy twist that contrasts with the sweetness of passionfruit.

**2. Mango Tango Fusion:**
   - Introduce the tropical allure of mango by adding a splash of mango puree to the mix.

**3. Coconut Hibiscus Bliss:**
   - Elevate the margarita with a splash of coconut cream for a creamy and exotic touch.

**4. Cucumber Serenity Splash:**
   - Muddle cucumber slices in the shaker for a refreshing and cooling element.

Feel free to explore these variations or craft your own signature twist on the Passion Hibiscus Margarita. Whether sipped by the beach or shared among friends, this tropical delight promises a taste of paradise in every festive moment. Cheers to the art of crafting vibrant and flavorful cocktails!

# Coconut Hibiscus Mojito: A Tropical Oasis in a Glass

Escape to a serene tropical oasis with the Coconut Hibiscus Mojito, a refreshing blend of coconut rum, vibrant hibiscus syrup, muddled mint leaves, zesty lime wedges, and a splash of invigorating soda water. This mojito is a symphony of flavors that transports you to a paradisiacal getaway with every sip.

## Ingredients:

- 2 oz coconut rum
- 1 oz hibiscus syrup
- 8-10 fresh mint leaves
- 1 lime, cut into wedges
- Soda water
- Ice cubes
- Hibiscus petal and mint sprig for garnish

## Instructions:

1. Prepare Hibiscus Syrup:
   - Create hibiscus syrup by combining hibiscus tea with an equal amount of sugar. Allow it to cool before use.

2. Muddle Mint and Lime:
   - In a glass, muddle fresh mint leaves and lime wedges to release their flavors.

3. Add Coconut Rum and Hibiscus Syrup:
   - Pour coconut rum and hibiscus syrup into the glass with the muddled mint and lime.

4. Shake or Stir:
   - If desired, gently shake the mixture with ice in a cocktail shaker, or stir it well to combine the ingredients.

5. Strain into Glass:
   - Strain the mixture into a highball glass filled with ice cubes.

6. Top with Soda Water:
   - Top the Coconut Hibiscus Mojito with soda water for a light effervescence. Adjust the amount to your preferred level of fizziness.

7. Garnish Creatively:
   - Garnish with a hibiscus petal and a sprig of fresh mint for a visually appealing and aromatic touch.

8. Sip and Transport:
   - Transport yourself to a tropical paradise with each sip of the Coconut Hibiscus Mojito, a harmonious fusion of coconut, hibiscus, and mint.

## Variations:

1. Pineapple Coconut Bliss:
   - Include a splash of pineapple juice for an extra layer of tropical sweetness.

2. Ginger Infusion:
   - Infuse the hibiscus syrup with a hint of freshly grated ginger for a subtle warmth.

3. Passionfruit Elegance:
   - Add a splash of passionfruit puree for an exotic and fruity twist.

4. Blueberry Coconut Crush:
   - Muddle a handful of fresh blueberries along with the mint and lime for a burst of berry goodness.

Feel free to experiment with these variations or create your own to tailor the Coconut Hibiscus Mojito to your taste preferences. Whether enjoyed as a solo retreat or shared in the company of friends, this tropical mojito promises a taste of paradise in every sip. Cheers to the art of crafting refreshing and vibrant cocktails!

# Spicy Hibiscus Pineapple Punch: A Fiery Fiesta in Every Sip

Ignite your taste buds with the Spicy Hibiscus Pineapple Punch, a tantalizing concoction featuring jalapeño-infused tequila, vibrant hibiscus syrup, luscious pineapple juice, and a dash of chili powder for an extra kick. This punch is a fiery fiesta that promises to exhilarate your senses with its bold and spicy allure.

## Variations:

**1. Mango Tango Blaze:**
   - Amp up the tropical heat by adding a splash of mango puree to the punch.

**2. Cucumber Cool Down:**
   - Balance the spice with a few cucumber slices for a refreshing and cooling element.

**3. Ginger Zest Infusion:**
   - Infuse the hibiscus syrup with a hint of freshly grated ginger for an additional layer of warmth.

**4. Smoky Chipotle Elevation:**
   - Substitute chili powder with a pinch of smoked chipotle powder for a smoky and intense flavor.

## Ingredients:

- 2 oz jalapeño-infused tequila
- 1 oz hibiscus syrup
- 3 oz pineapple juice
- Dash of chili powder
- Ice cubes
- Jalapeño slice for garnish (optional)
- Pineapple wedge for garnish

## Instructions:

**1. Prepare Jalapeño-Infused Tequila:**
   - Infuse tequila with slices of jalapeño. Allow it to steep for at least 24 hours, then strain to obtain jalapeño-infused tequila.

**2. Combine Ingredients:**
   - In a shaker, combine jalapeño-infused tequila, hibiscus syrup, and pineapple juice.

**3. Shake Vigorously:**
   - Shake the mixture with ice vigorously to infuse the flavors and chill the punch.

**4. Strain into Glass:**
   - Strain the punch into a highball glass filled with ice cubes.

**5. Dash of Chili Powder:**
   - Add a dash of chili powder to the top of the punch for a spicy and smoky dimension. Adjust the amount to your desired level of heat.

**6. Garnish Creatively:**
   - Garnish with a jalapeño slice for an extra kick (optional) and a pineapple wedge for a tropical touch.

**7. Stir Gently:**
   - Optionally, give the punch a gentle stir to incorporate the chili powder into the mix.

**8. Sip and Savor the Heat:**
   - Dive into the Spicy Hibiscus Pineapple Punch and relish the bold and fiery fusion of jalapeño, hibiscus, and pineapple.

# Blue Lagoon Hibiscus Fizz: A Breathtaking Burst of Color and Flavor

Immerse yourself in the stunning beauty of the Blue Lagoon Hibiscus Fizz, a mesmerizing concoction that combines the vibrant hues of Blue Curaçao with the floral notes of hibiscus-infused gin, zesty lemon juice, and the effervescence of soda water. This fizz is not only a visual spectacle but also a delightful journey for your taste buds.

## Variations:

**1. Tropical Paradise Twist:**
- Enhance the tropical vibes by adding a splash of pineapple juice to the mix.

**2. Minty Blue Oasis:**
- Muddle a few fresh mint leaves in the shaker for a burst of herbal freshness.

**3. Vanilla Hibiscus Elegance:**
- Float a few drops of vanilla extract on the surface for a subtle sweetness that complements the floral hibiscus.

**4. Ginger Hibiscus Burst:**
- Infuse the hibiscus syrup with a hint of freshly grated ginger for an extra layer of warmth.

## Ingredients:

- 1 1/2 oz Blue Curaçao
- 1 oz hibiscus-infused gin
- 3/4 oz fresh lemon juice
- Soda water
- Ice cubes
- Lemon wheel for garnish
- Edible flowers (optional) for an artistic touch

## Instructions:

**1. Prepare Hibiscus-Infused Gin:**
- Infuse gin with dried hibiscus petals. Allow it to steep for at least 24 hours, then strain to obtain hibiscus-infused gin.

**2. Combine Ingredients:**
- In a shaker, combine Blue Curaçao, hibiscus-infused gin, and fresh lemon juice.

**3. Shake Well:**
- Shake the mixture with ice vigorously to chill and blend the flavors.

**4. Strain into Glass:**
- Strain the vibrant mixture into a highball or Collins glass filled with ice cubes.

**5. Top with Soda Water:**
- Top the Blue Lagoon Hibiscus Fizz with soda water for a lively effervescence. Adjust the amount to your preferred level of fizziness.

**6. Garnish Creatively:**
- Garnish with a lemon wheel for a citrusy aroma and, if available, edible flowers for a touch of artistry.

**7. Stir Gently:**
- Optionally, give the fizz a gentle stir to incorporate the soda water into the mix.

**8. Sip and Dive In:**
- Dive into the visually stunning Blue Lagoon Hibiscus Fizz and savor the harmonious blend of colors and flavors.

# Mango Habanero Hibiscus Splash: A Spicy Tropical Symphony

Embark on a spicy and tropical journey with the Mango Habanero Hibiscus Splash, a captivating concoction that blends the lusciousness of mango vodka, the floral notes of hibiscus-infused rum, the fiery kick of habanero syrup, and the citrusy brightness of orange juice. This splash is a symphony of flavors that promises to tantalize your taste buds with every sip.

## Variations:

### 1. Coconut Heat Wave:
- Elevate the tropical essence by adding a splash of coconut cream for a creamy and exotic touch.

### 2. Pineapple Passion Blaze:
- Infuse the splash with the tropical sweetness of pineapple juice for an extra layer of fruity goodness.

### 3. Minty Firestorm:
- Muddle a few fresh mint leaves in the shaker for a cooling and herbal contrast to the heat.

### 4. Vanilla Heat Elegance:
- Float a few drops of vanilla extract on the surface for a touch of sweetness that complements the spiciness.

## Ingredients:

- 1 1/2 oz Mango Vodka
- 1 oz hibiscus-infused rum
- 1/2 oz habanero syrup
- 2 oz orange juice
- Ice cubes
- Habanero slice for garnish (optional)
- Mango slice for garnish

## Instructions:

1. **Prepare Hibiscus-Infused Rum:**
   - Infuse rum with dried hibiscus petals. Allow it to steep for at least 24 hours, then strain to obtain hibiscus-infused rum.

2. **Prepare Habanero Syrup:**
   - Create habanero syrup by combining equal parts water and sugar, then infuse it with sliced habanero peppers. Strain the syrup to remove the pepper slices.

3. **Combine Ingredients:**
   - In a shaker, combine mango vodka, hibiscus-infused rum, habanero syrup, and orange juice.

4. **Shake Vigorously:**
   - Shake the mixture with ice vigorously to infuse the flavors and chill the splash.

5. **Strain into Glass:**
   - Strain the vibrant Mango Habanero Hibiscus Splash into a highball glass filled with ice cubes.

6. **Garnish Creatively:**
   - Garnish with a slice of habanero for an extra spicy kick (optional) and a mango slice for a tropical flourish.

7. **Stir Gently:**
   - Optionally, give the splash a gentle stir to combine the ingredients.

8. **Sip and Savor the Heat:**
   - Savor the Mango Habanero Hibiscus Splash, a spicy and tropical symphony that dances on your palate with each sip.

# Cucumber Basil Hibiscus Sling: A Refreshing Botanical Symphony

Embark on a journey of refreshing botanicals with the Cucumber Basil Hibiscus Sling, a sophisticated concoction featuring the classic touch of gin, the floral allure of hibiscus liqueur, the crispness of cucumber slices, the aromatic notes of basil leaves, and the effervescence of tonic. This sling is a harmonious symphony of flavors that invites you to savor the crisp and revitalizing essence of its botanical blend.

## Variations:

**1. Citrus Burst Elevation:**
- Enhance the sling with a squeeze of fresh lime or lemon juice for a citrusy twist.

**2. Minty Cucumber Oasis:**
- Muddle a few fresh mint leaves in the shaker for a cooling and herbal element.

**3. Ginger Basil Zest:**
- Infuse the hibiscus liqueur with a hint of freshly grated ginger for an extra layer of warmth.

**4. Vanilla Basil Infusion:**
- Float a few drops of vanilla extract on the surface for a subtle sweetness that complements the botanicals.

## Ingredients:

- 2 oz Gin
- 1 oz Hibiscus Liqueur
- Cucumber slices
- Basil leaves
- Tonic water
- Ice cubes
- Basil sprig and cucumber ribbon for garnish

## Instructions:

**1. Prepare Cucumber Infusion:**
- Infuse gin with cucumber slices by letting them steep in the gin for at least 30 minutes.

**2. Combine Ingredients:**
- In a shaker, combine the cucumber-infused gin and hibiscus liqueur.

**3. Add Fresh Basil and Ice:**
- Drop a few fresh basil leaves into the shaker and add ice cubes.

**4. Shake Gently:**
- Give the mixture a gentle shake to incorporate the flavors and chill the ingredients.

**5. Strain into Glass:**
- Strain the infused mixture into a highball glass filled with ice cubes.

**6. Top with Tonic Water:**
- Top the Cucumber Basil Hibiscus Sling with tonic water to add a refreshing effervescence. Adjust the amount to your preferred level of fizziness.

**7. Garnish Creatively:**
- Garnish with a basil sprig for a burst of aroma and a cucumber ribbon for an elegant visual touch.

**8. Stir Gently:**
- Optionally, give the sling a gentle stir to combine the tonic water with the infused mixture.

# Hibiscus Paloma: A Floral Citrus Symphony

Indulge in the vibrant and floral notes of the Hibiscus Paloma, a delightful concoction featuring the allure of hibiscus-infused tequila, the citrusy brightness of grapefruit juice, the natural sweetness of agave syrup, and the effervescence of club soda. This Paloma is a refreshing symphony that promises to transport your taste buds to a sun-soaked paradise with every sip.

## Variations:

**1. Spicy Hibiscus Twist:**
 - Add a slice of jalapeño to the shaker for a spicy kick that contrasts with the floral and citrus notes.

**2. Mango Hibiscus Fusion:**
 - Include a splash of mango puree for an additional layer of tropical sweetness.

**3. Basil Hibiscus Breeze:**
 - Infuse the hibiscus syrup with fresh basil leaves for an herbal undertone.

**4. Vanilla Citrus Elegance:**
 - Float a few drops of vanilla extract on the surface for a subtle sweetness that complements the floral hibiscus.

## Ingredients:

- 2 oz Hibiscus-Infused Tequila
- 3 oz Grapefruit Juice
- 1/2 oz Agave Syrup
- Club Soda
- Ice cubes
- Grapefruit wedge for garnish
- Hibiscus petal for garnish

## Instructions:

**1. Prepare Hibiscus-Infused Tequila:**
 - Infuse tequila with dried hibiscus petals. Allow it to steep for at least 24 hours, then strain to obtain hibiscus-infused tequila.

**2. Combine Ingredients:**
 - In a shaker, combine hibiscus-infused tequila, grapefruit juice, and agave syrup.

**3. Shake Well:**
 - Shake the mixture with ice vigorously to blend the flavors and chill the Paloma.

**4. Strain into Glass:**
 - Strain the vibrant mixture into a highball glass filled with ice cubes.

**5. Top with Club Soda:**
 - Top the Hibiscus Paloma with club soda for a refreshing effervescence. Adjust the amount to your preferred level of fizziness.

**6. Garnish Creatively:**
 - Garnish with a grapefruit wedge for a citrusy aroma and a hibiscus petal for a touch of floral elegance.

**7. Stir Gently:**
 - Optionally, give the Paloma a gentle stir to combine the club soda with the infused mixture.

**8. Sip and Transport:**
 - Immerse yourself in the floral citrus symphony of the Hibiscus Paloma, a refreshing escape in every sip.

## Smoky Hibiscus Mezcal Mule: A Fiery Elixir with Floral Undertones

Experience the bold and smoky allure of the Smoky Hibiscus Mezcal Mule, a fiery elixir that combines the robust flavor of mezcal with the floral notes of hibiscus syrup, the zesty kick of lime juice, and the effervescence of ginger beer. To enhance the smoky profile, the glass is elegantly rimmed with a smoky salt, adding an extra layer of complexity to this invigorating mule.

### Variations:

**1. Spicy Smoky Sensation:**
- Infuse the hibiscus syrup with a slice of jalapeño for an additional spicy kick.

**2. Pineapple Hibiscus Blaze:**
- Add a splash of pineapple juice to the mix for a tropical and fruity twist.

**3. Cinnamon Smoke Infusion:**
- Infuse the mezcal with a cinnamon stick for a warm and aromatic undertone.

**4. Vanilla Hibiscus Harmony:**
- Float a few drops of vanilla extract on the surface for a subtle sweetness that complements the floral hibiscus.

### Ingredients:

- 2 oz Mezcal
- 1 oz Hibiscus Syrup
- 3/4 oz Lime Juice
- Ginger Beer
- Smoky Salt (for rimming)
- Ice cubes
- Lime wheel for garnish
- Hibiscus petal for garnish

### Instructions:

**1. Rim the Glass with Smoky Salt:**
- Moisten the rim of a copper mug or highball glass with a lime wedge, then dip it into smoky salt to coat the rim.

**2. Combine Ingredients:**
- In the prepared glass, combine mezcal, hibiscus syrup, and lime juice.

**3. Add Ice Cubes:**
- Fill the glass with ice cubes to chill the mixture.

**4. Top with Ginger Beer:**
- Top the Smoky Hibiscus Mezcal Mule with ginger beer, adjusting the amount to your preferred level of effervescence.

**5. Garnish Creatively:**
- Garnish with a lime wheel for a citrusy aroma and a hibiscus petal for an elegant touch.

**6. Stir Gently:**
- Optionally, give the mule a gentle stir to combine the flavors.

**7. Sip and Savor the Smoky Elegance:**
- Delight in the robust and smoky elegance of the Smoky Hibiscus Mezcal Mule, a fiery elixir with floral undertones.

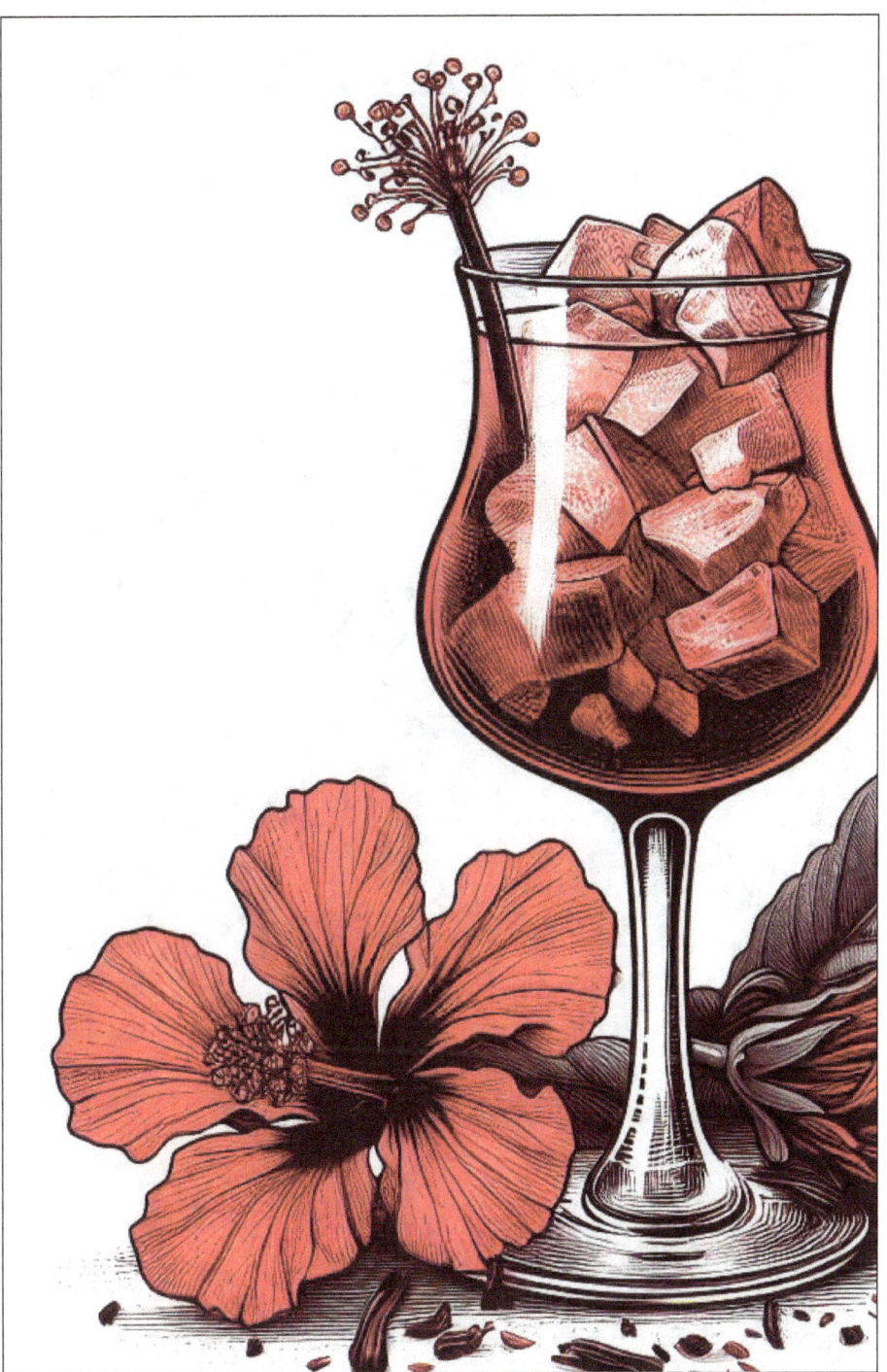

# Tinctures and Elixirs

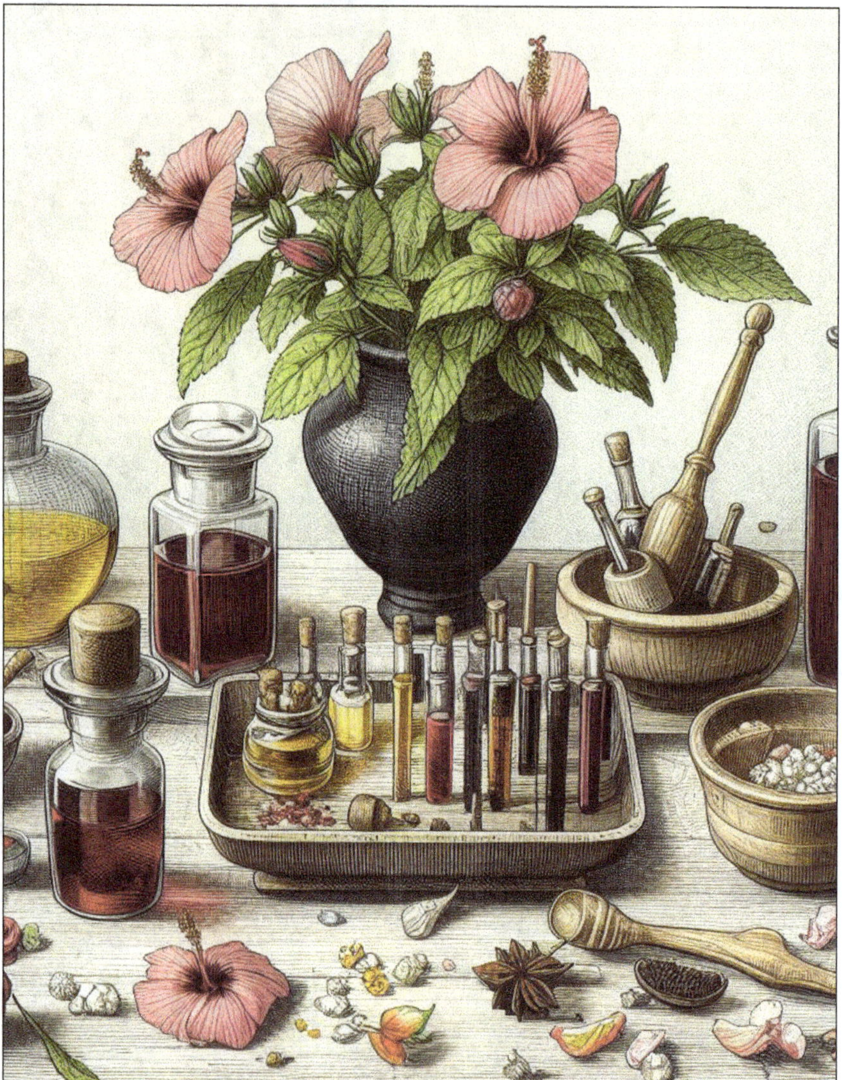

## History:
Tinctures and elixirs have a rich history dating back centuries. The practice of using alcohol or other solvents to extract and preserve the medicinal properties of plants is ancient and spans various cultures. Traditional herbal medicine systems, including Ayurveda, Traditional Chinese Medicine (TCM), and Western herbalism, have incorporated tinctures and elixirs for their therapeutic benefits.

## Uses:
**1. Traditional Medicine:**
- Tinctures and elixirs are staples in traditional medicine systems worldwide, addressing various health concerns such as digestive issues, respiratory ailments, and stress.

**2. Naturopathy:**
- Naturopaths often employ tinctures and elixirs as part of a holistic approach to health, considering the individual's overall well-being.

**3. Folk Medicine:**
- In folk medicine, these preparations are used for a wide range of conditions, passed down through generations based on experiential knowledge.

**4. Medical Studies:**
- Some herbs used in tinctures and elixirs have undergone scientific scrutiny. While research supports the efficacy of certain herbs, more studies are needed to establish conclusive evidence.

## Procedures:
**1. Extraction Process:**
- Tinctures involve extracting active compounds from herbs using alcohol or another solvent. Elixirs typically include sweeteners and additional herbs for flavor.

**2. Maceration:**
- The maceration process involves soaking herbs in alcohol for an extended period, allowing the solvent to extract the medicinal constituents.

**3. Filtration:**
- After maceration, the mixture is often filtered to remove plant material, resulting in a concentrated liquid.

## Contemporary Uses:
**1. Health Supplements:**
- Tinctures and elixirs are available as health supplements in modern herbalism, catering to individuals seeking natural remedies.

**2. Holistic Health Practices:**
- They are integrated into holistic health practices, aligning with the growing interest in natural and alternative therapies.

## Warnings:
**1. Alcohol Content:**
- Tinctures may contain high alcohol content, which can be a concern for individuals avoiding alcohol or those with certain health conditions.

**2. Dosage Accuracy:**
- Accurate dosing is crucial. Improperly prepared tinctures or elixirs may result in inconsistent or potentially harmful dosages.

**3. Interactions:**
- Herb-drug interactions are possible. Individuals on medications should consult healthcare professionals to avoid adverse effects.

**4. Quality Control:**
- The quality of the herbs and the extraction process impact efficacy. Purchasing from reputable sources is essential.

**Disclaimer:**

The information provided here is for educational and informational purposes only and should not be considered as professional medical advice. Herbal remedies and homemade treatments carry potential risks and may not be suitable for everyone. It is crucial to consult with a qualified healthcare professional or herbalist before attempting any herbal remedies, especially if you are pregnant, nursing, taking medications, or have any underlying health conditions.

Individuals may react differently to herbs, and what works for one person may not be suitable for another. It is essential to perform patch tests before using any herbal products topically to avoid potential allergic reactions. Additionally, herbal remedies should not be used as a substitute for professional medical diagnosis or treatment.

The content provided does not intend to diagnose, treat, cure, or prevent any disease. Always seek the advice of your physician or other qualified health provider with any questions you may have regarding a medical condition. Never disregard professional medical advice or delay in seeking it because of information provided in this response.

By engaging in the use of herbal remedies, you acknowledge that you do so at your own risk, and you are responsible for ensuring the safety and appropriateness of the remedies for your individual health needs.

**Consulting a Professional:**

To consult with a licensed herbalist or naturopath in the U.S., individuals can follow a systematic approach to ensure the quality and safety of the services received. Firstly, it is advisable to verify the practitioner's credentials by checking their licensure and certifications. In the United States, herbalists may hold certifications from recognized organizations or have completed formal education in herbal medicine. For naturopaths, confirming that the practitioner is licensed in their state is essential, as licensure requirements can vary.

Potential clients can seek recommendations from healthcare professionals, friends, or family who have had positive experiences with herbalists or naturopaths. Additionally, researching online reviews and testimonials can provide insights into the practitioner's reputation. Prior to scheduling an appointment, individuals should prepare a list of questions, including inquiries about the practitioner's approach to herbal medicine, treatment plans, and any relevant experience with specific health concerns. During the consultation, open communication is key.

Clients should be transparent about their medical history, current medications, and any ongoing treatments to facilitate a comprehensive and personalized herbal or naturopathic approach. Importantly, individuals should discuss the integration of herbal remedies with any existing medical treatments and seek collaboration between the herbalist or naturopath and their primary healthcare provider. This collaborative approach ensures that the care received aligns with the individual's overall health and well-being.

**Wise Use Advice:**

It is essential to exercise caution and consider potential interactions when using herbal remedies, especially if you are already taking medications or substances that may impact your health. Here are some general pieces of advice:

1. Alcohol:
   - Alcohol can enhance the sedative effects of certain herbs and may interact with the compounds in the elixirs. It's advisable to avoid consuming alcohol when using herbal tinctures, especially those with relaxing or sedative properties.

2. Marijuana (Cannabis):
   - Cannabis may have varying effects when combined with herbal remedies. While some combinations could be synergistic, others might lead to unwanted side effects. It's recommended to approach such combinations with caution and, if possible, consult with a healthcare professional.

3. Depressive Drugs (Antidepressants):
   - Some herbs used in these elixirs may have interactions with antidepressant medications. For instance, St. John's Wort, an herb known for its mood-boosting properties, can interact with certain antidepressants. If you are on antidepressant medication, consult with your healthcare provider before using herbal remedies.

4. Prescription Medications:
   - Always consult with your healthcare provider before incorporating herbal remedies into your routine, especially if you are taking prescription medications. Some herbs may interact with medications, affecting their effectiveness or leading to undesirable side effects.

5. Individual Health Conditions:
   - If you have pre-existing health conditions, allergies, or concerns about interactions, it's crucial to seek advice from a healthcare professional. They can provide personalized guidance based on your medical history.

6. Pregnancy and Breastfeeding:
   - Pregnant and breastfeeding individuals should exercise caution with herbal remedies. Some herbs may have contraindications during pregnancy or lactation. Always consult with a healthcare provider before using herbal products during these periods.

7. Individual Reactions:
   - Individuals can react differently to herbs. Monitor your body's response, and if you experience any adverse effects or discomfort, discontinue use and seek medical advice.

8. Professional Guidance:
   - When in doubt, seek guidance from a qualified healthcare professional or herbalist. They can provide personalized advice based on your health status and help you navigate potential interactions.

Remember, herbal remedies should be viewed as complementary to, not a replacement for, conventional medical care. Always communicate openly with your healthcare provider about any herbal supplements you are considering to ensure a safe and well-informed approach to your health.

## Hibiscus Heart Health Elixir

This elixir combines hibiscus, hawthorn, and motherwort, renowned herbs for cardiovascular support.

### Ingredients:

- 2 tablespoons dried hibiscus petals
- 1 tablespoon dried hawthorn berries
- 1 tablespoon dried motherwort leaves
- 1 cinnamon stick
- 1-2 teaspoons raw honey (optional, for sweetness)
- 2 cups filtered water

### Instructions:

1. Prepare the Herbs:
   - In a teapot or heat-resistant container, combine the dried hibiscus petals, hawthorn berries, motherwort leaves, and a cinnamon stick.

2. Boil Water:
   - Heat 2 cups of filtered water until it reaches a gentle boil.

3. Infuse the Herbs:
   - Pour the hot water over the herbs in the teapot. Cover and let it steep for about 15-20 minutes.

4. Strain the Elixir:
   - After steeping, strain the elixir to remove the herbs. Use a fine mesh strainer or cheesecloth to ensure a clear liquid.

5. Sweeten (Optional):
   - If desired, add 1-2 teaspoons of raw honey to the elixir and stir until dissolved. Adjust the sweetness to your preference.

6. Serve and Enjoy:
   - Pour the elixir into cups or mugs. Sip and savor the herbal infusion.

### Hibiscus Heart Health Elixir History:

The use of hibiscus, hawthorn, and motherwort in herbal medicine for cardiovascular support has historical roots in various traditional healing systems.

- **Hibiscus:** Known for its vibrant red flowers, hibiscus has been used in traditional medicine globally. Rich in antioxidants and anthocyanins, hibiscus is believed to support heart health by promoting healthy blood pressure levels.

- **Hawthorn:** A staple in Western herbalism, hawthorn has a long history of use for heart-related conditions. It is thought to enhance cardiovascular function, improve blood flow, and support overall heart health.

- **Motherwort:** Widely used in Traditional Chinese Medicine (TCM) and European herbalism, motherwort is valued for its calming properties and potential benefits for heart health. It is believed to promote circulation and ease heart palpitations.

Combining these herbs in an elixir creates a synergistic blend, offering a delightful and therapeutic beverage. As with any herbal remedy, it's advisable to consult with a healthcare professional, especially if you have pre-existing medical conditions or are on medication.

## Digestive Hibiscus Bitters Recipe

Bitters are herbal extracts known for their digestive benefits. Hibiscus adds a unique and flavorful twist to this digestive bitters recipe.

**Ingredients:**

- 1/4 cup dried hibiscus petals
- 1 tablespoon dried chamomile flowers
- 1 tablespoon dried orange peel
- 1 tablespoon dried ginger root
- 1 tablespoon dried dandelion root
- 1 tablespoon dried fennel seeds
- 1 tablespoon dried mint leaves
- 1 cinnamon stick
- 1 cup high-proof alcohol (e.g., vodka or brandy)
- 1/2 cup water
- 1-2 tablespoons honey (optional, for sweetness)

**Instructions:**

1. Combine Herbs:
   - In a glass jar with a tight-fitting lid, combine the dried hibiscus petals, chamomile flowers, orange peel, ginger root, dandelion root, fennel seeds, mint leaves, and cinnamon stick.

2. Add Alcohol:
   - Pour the high-proof alcohol over the herbs in the jar. Ensure that the herbs are completely submerged. The alcohol acts as a solvent to extract the medicinal properties of the herbs.

3. Maceration:
   - Seal the jar tightly and place it in a cool, dark place for about 2-4 weeks. Shake the jar every few days to encourage the maceration process.

4. Strain the Mixture:
   - After the maceration period, strain the liquid through a fine mesh strainer or cheesecloth into a clean bowl or jar. Squeeze the herbs to extract any remaining liquid.

5. Prepare Simple Syrup:
   - In a saucepan, heat 1/2 cup of water. If you prefer a sweeter bitters, add 1-2 tablespoons of honey to the water and stir until dissolved. Allow the simple syrup to cool.

6. Combine and Adjust:
   - Combine the strained herbal extract with the simple syrup. Taste the mixture and adjust sweetness if necessary.

7. Bottle and Store:
   - Pour the digestive hibiscus bitters into dark glass bottles with dropper lids. Store the bottles in a cool, dark place.

8. Usage:
   - To support digestion, take 1-2 dropperfuls of the bitters before meals. You can dilute it in a small amount of water if desired.

## Enhanced Pacific Island Digestive Tincture

Embark on a sensory journey with our Enhanced Pacific Island Digestive Tincture, a fusion of vibrant herbs from the Pacific Rim. This exquisite elixir is a harmonious blend of traditional Pacific Island digestive allies and additional treasures from Southeast Asia, creating a tapestry of flavors and potential wellness benefits.

### Ingredients:

- 2 tablespoons dried hibiscus petals
- 1 tablespoon dried ginger root
- 1 tablespoon dried lemongrass
- 1 teaspoon fennel seeds
- 1 teaspoon dried mint leaves
- 1 teaspoon dried kaffir lime leaves
- 1 teaspoon dried pandan leaves
- 1 teaspoon dried turmeric slices
- 1 cup high-proof alcohol (e.g., vodka or rum)

### Instructions:

1. Prepare the Herbs:
   - In a clean glass jar with a tight-fitting lid, combine the dried hibiscus petals, dried ginger root, dried lemongrass, fennel seeds, dried mint leaves, dried kaffir lime leaves, dried pandan leaves, and dried turmeric slices.

2. Add Alcohol:
   - Pour the high-proof alcohol over the herbs, ensuring they are fully submerged. The alcohol acts as a solvent to extract the active compounds.

3. Maceration:
   - Seal the jar tightly and place it in a cool, dark place for 4-6 weeks. Shake the jar gently every few days to facilitate the maceration process.

4. Strain the Tincture:
   - After the maceration period, strain the liquid through a fine mesh strainer or cheesecloth into a clean glass container. Squeeze the herbs to extract any remaining liquid.

5. Bottle and Store:
   - Transfer the strained tincture into dark glass bottles with dropper lids. Store the bottles in a cool, dark place.

6. Usage:
   - Start with a small dose, such as 1/2 to 1 dropperful, before or after meals to aid in digestion. Adjust the dosage as needed.

### Pacific Rim Ingredients:

- **Kaffir Lime Leaves:**
  - Kaffir lime leaves contribute a citrusy and floral aroma, commonly used in Southeast Asian cuisine. They add a unique twist to the tincture.

- **Pandan Leaves:**
  - Pandan leaves impart a sweet and nutty flavor, frequently used in Pacific Rim desserts. They can add a delightful complexity to the tincture.

- **Turmeric:**
  - Turmeric brings its earthy and slightly bitter notes to the tincture, along with potential anti-inflammatory properties.

Feel free to adjust the proportions based on your taste preferences, and enjoy this enhanced Pacific Island Digestive Tincture as a flavorful and digestive-supportive addition to your wellness routine. As always, consult with a healthcare professional, especially if you have specific health concerns or are taking medications.

# Hibiscus Hormonal Balance Tincture Recipe

This tincture combines hibiscus, vitex (chaste tree), and dong quai, known for their potential to support hormonal balance.

## Hibiscus Hormonal Balance Tincture Background:

- **Hibiscus:** Renowned for its vibrant flowers, hibiscus is rich in antioxidants and may contribute to overall well-being. In this tincture, hibiscus adds both flavor and potential health benefits.

- **Vitex (Chaste Tree):** Vitex has a long history of use in supporting female hormonal balance. It is commonly used to address menstrual irregularities and promote reproductive health.

- **Dong Quai:** Often referred to as the "female ginseng" in traditional Chinese medicine, dong quai is believed to have adaptogenic properties, supporting hormonal balance and menstrual health.

Combining these herbs in a tincture offers a convenient way to incorporate their potential benefits into daily wellness routines. As with any herbal remedy, it's advisable to consult with a healthcare professional, especially for individuals with hormonal imbalances, underlying health conditions, or those taking medications.

## Ingredients:

- 1/4 cup dried hibiscus petals
- 2 tablespoons dried vitex (chaste tree) berries
- 1 tablespoon dried dong quai root
- 1 cup high-proof alcohol (e.g., vodka or brandy)

## Instructions:

1. Prepare the Herbs:
   - In a clean glass jar with a tight-fitting lid, combine the dried hibiscus petals, vitex berries, and dong quai root.

2. Add Alcohol:
   - Pour the high-proof alcohol over the herbs, ensuring they are fully submerged. The alcohol acts as a solvent to extract the active compounds.

3. Maceration:
   - Seal the jar tightly and place it in a cool, dark place for 4-6 weeks. Shake the jar gently every few days to facilitate the maceration process.

4. Strain the Tincture:
   - After the maceration period, strain the liquid through a fine mesh strainer or cheesecloth into a clean glass container. Squeeze the herbs to extract any remaining liquid.

5. Bottle and Store:
   - Transfer the strained tincture into dark glass bottles with dropper lids. Store the bottles in a cool, dark place.

6. Usage:
   - Start with a small dose, such as 1/2 to 1 dropperful, and gradually increase if needed. Take the tincture once or twice daily, depending on individual preferences and needs.

## Hibiscus Immune Elixir

This immune-boosting elixir combines hibiscus with echinacea, elderberry, and other herbs known for their potential immune support.

Ingredients:

- 2 tablespoons dried hibiscus petals
- 1 tablespoon dried echinacea purpurea
- 1 tablespoon dried elderberries
- 1 tablespoon dried astragalus root
- 1 tablespoon dried rose hips
- 1 cinnamon stick
- 1 cup high-proof alcohol (e.g., vodka or brandy) or honey for a syrup option
- 1/2 cup water (for syrup option)

Instructions:

1. Prepare the Herbs:
   - In a clean glass jar, combine the dried hibiscus petals, echinacea, elderberries, astragalus root, rose hips, and a cinnamon stick.

2. Choose Extraction Method:
   - For a tincture, pour the high-proof alcohol over the herbs, ensuring they are fully submerged. For a syrup, bring water to a gentle boil, add honey, and stir until dissolved. Pour the honey-water mixture over the herbs.

3. Maceration or Infusion:
   - Seal the jar tightly and place it in a cool, dark place for 4-6 weeks for a tincture. If making a syrup, allow the herbs to infuse in the honey-water mixture for a few hours or overnight.

4. Strain the Elixir:
   - After the maceration or infusion period, strain the liquid through a fine mesh strainer or cheesecloth into a clean glass container. Squeeze the herbs to extract any remaining liquid.

5. Bottle and Store:
   - Transfer the strained elixir into dark glass bottles with dropper lids for the tincture or a glass jar for the syrup. Store in a cool, dark place.

6. Usage:
   - For the tincture, take 1 dropperful once or twice daily, adjusting as needed. For the syrup, take 1-2 teaspoons daily. Dilute in water or tea if desired.

Hibiscus Immune Elixir History and Contraindications:

- **History:**
   - Hibiscus, echinacea, elderberry, astragalus, and rose hips have historical roots in traditional medicine systems globally. They are revered for their immune-boosting properties and have been used for centuries to support overall wellness.

- **Contraindications:**
   - While these herbs are generally considered safe, individuals with autoimmune conditions or those on immunosuppressive medications should consult with a healthcare professional before using immune-boosting supplements. Additionally, pregnant or breastfeeding individuals should seek guidance from a healthcare provider before incorporating such elixirs into their routine.

This elixir offers a delightful and potentially beneficial way to support immune health. As with any herbal remedy, it's essential to approach it with individual considerations and consult with a healthcare professional, especially for those with specific health conditions or concerns.

## Hibiscus Joint Relief Elixir

This elixir blends hibiscus with turmeric and ginger, known for their anti-inflammatory properties, creating a tincture aimed at supporting joint health.

### Ingredients:

- 2 tablespoons dried hibiscus petals
- 1 tablespoon dried turmeric root (sliced or grated)
- 1 tablespoon fresh ginger root (sliced or grated)
- 1 teaspoon black pepper (enhances turmeric absorption)
- 1 cup high-proof alcohol (e.g., vodka or brandy)

### Instructions:

1. Prepare the Herbs:
   - In a clean glass jar with a tight-fitting lid, combine the dried hibiscus petals, dried turmeric root, fresh ginger root, and black pepper.

2. Add Alcohol:
   - Pour the high-proof alcohol over the herbs, ensuring they are fully submerged. The alcohol serves as a solvent to extract the active compounds.

3. Maceration:
   - Seal the jar tightly and place it in a cool, dark place for 4-6 weeks. Shake the jar gently every few days to facilitate the maceration process.

4. Strain the Tincture:
   - After the maceration period, strain the liquid through a fine mesh strainer or cheesecloth into a clean glass container. Squeeze the herbs to extract any remaining liquid.

5. Bottle and Store:
   - Transfer the strained tincture into dark glass bottles with dropper lids. Store the bottles in a cool, dark place.

6. Usage:
   - Start with a small dose, such as 1/2 to 1 dropperful, and gradually increase if needed. Take the tincture once or twice daily, depending on individual preferences and needs.

### Hibiscus Joint Relief Elixir Background:

- **Hibiscus:** Rich in antioxidants, hibiscus may contribute to overall well-being. In this elixir, hibiscus adds a flavorful and vibrant element.

- **Turmeric:** Known for its active compound curcumin, turmeric has potent anti-inflammatory properties that may help alleviate joint discomfort.

- **Ginger:** Ginger has anti-inflammatory and antioxidant effects, potentially providing relief from joint pain and stiffness.

- **Black Pepper:** Contains piperine, enhancing the bioavailability of curcumin from turmeric, optimizing its benefits.

Combining these herbs in a tincture offers a convenient way to incorporate their potential joint-supportive properties. As with any herbal remedy, it's advisable to consult with a healthcare professional, especially for individuals with joint issues, underlying health conditions, or those taking medications.

## Hibiscus Respiratory Tincture

This respiratory tincture combines hibiscus with thyme and mullein, herbs known for their potential respiratory health benefits.

Ingredients:

- 2 tablespoons dried hibiscus petals
- 1 tablespoon dried thyme leaves
- 1 tablespoon dried mullein leaves
- 1 cup high-proof alcohol (e.g., vodka or brandy)

Instructions:

1. Prepare the Herbs:
   - In a clean glass jar with a tight-fitting lid, combine the dried hibiscus petals, dried thyme leaves, and dried mullein leaves.

2. Add Alcohol:
   - Pour the high-proof alcohol over the herbs, ensuring they are fully submerged. The alcohol acts as a solvent to extract the active compounds.

3. Maceration:
   - Seal the jar tightly and place it in a cool, dark place for 4-6 weeks. Shake the jar gently every few days to facilitate the maceration process.

4. Strain the Tincture:
   - After the maceration period, strain the liquid through a fine mesh strainer or cheesecloth into a clean glass container. Squeeze the herbs to extract any remaining liquid.

5. Bottle and Store:
   - Transfer the strained tincture into dark glass bottles with dropper lids. Store the bottles in a cool, dark place.

6. Usage:
   - Start with a small dose, such as 1/2 to 1 dropperful, and gradually increase if needed. Take the tincture once or twice daily, depending on individual preferences and respiratory needs.

### Hibiscus Respiratory Tincture Background:

- **Hibiscus:** Rich in antioxidants, hibiscus may contribute to overall well-being. In this tincture, hibiscus adds a flavorful and vibrant element.

- **Thyme:** Known for its antimicrobial and expectorant properties, thyme has been used traditionally to support respiratory health.

- **Mullein:** Recognized for its soothing properties, mullein is often used to help alleviate respiratory discomfort and promote overall lung health.

Combining these herbs in a tincture offers a convenient way to incorporate their potential respiratory-supportive properties. As with any herbal remedy, it's advisable to consult with a healthcare professional, especially for individuals with respiratory concerns, underlying health conditions, or those taking medications.

## Hibiscus Sleep Aid Elixir

This sleep aid elixir combines hibiscus with calming herbs to promote relaxation and better sleep.

### Ingredients:

- 2 tablespoons dried hibiscus petals
- 1 tablespoon dried chamomile flowers
- 1 tablespoon dried passionflower
- 1 tablespoon dried lavender buds
- 1 teaspoon dried valerian root (optional, for added relaxation)
- 1 cup hot water
- 1-2 teaspoons raw honey (optional, for sweetness)

### Instructions:

1. Prepare the Herbs:
   - In a teapot or heat-resistant container, combine the dried hibiscus petals, chamomile flowers, passionflower, lavender buds, and valerian root (if using).

2. Infuse the Herbs:
   - Pour hot water over the herbs in the teapot. Cover and let it steep for about 10-15 minutes.

3. Strain the Elixir:
   - After steeping, strain the liquid through a fine mesh strainer or tea infuser into a clean mug or teacup.

4. Sweeten (Optional):
   - If desired, add 1-2 teaspoons of raw honey to the elixir and stir until dissolved. Adjust sweetness to your preference.

5. Sip and Enjoy:
   - Sip the elixir slowly about 30 minutes before bedtime to promote relaxation and a restful night's sleep.

### Hibiscus Sleep Aid Elixir Contraindications:

- **Valerian Root:** While valerian root is generally considered safe, it may cause drowsiness, so avoid operating machinery or driving after consuming it. Pregnant and breastfeeding individuals should consult with a healthcare professional before using valerian.

- **Passionflower:** Passionflower is generally safe for most people, but it may cause drowsiness. Avoid combining it with sedative medications, and pregnant or breastfeeding individuals should consult with a healthcare professional.

- **Individual Allergies:** Individuals with allergies to plants in the Asteraceae family (such as chamomile) should exercise caution.

It's crucial to consult with a healthcare professional before incorporating new herbs into your routine, especially if you are pregnant, breastfeeding, have pre-existing health conditions, or are taking medications. This sleep aid elixir is not a substitute for professional medical advice, diagnosis, or treatment.

## Hibiscus Lavender Sleep Elixir

This Hibiscus Lavender Sleep Elixir is a delightful infusion of soothing herbs designed to promote relaxation and facilitate a restful night's sleep. The bright and tangy notes of hibiscus are complemented by the gentle floral tones of lavender, creating a fragrant elixir that engages the senses. Chamomile and lemon balm contribute their calming properties, making this elixir a comforting and aromatic bedtime ritual.

### Ingredients:

- 2 tablespoons dried hibiscus petals
- 1 tablespoon dried lavender buds
- 1 teaspoon dried chamomile flowers
- 1 teaspoon dried lemon balm leaves
- 1 cup hot water
- 1-2 teaspoons raw honey (optional, for sweetness)

### Instructions:

1. Prepare the Herbs:
   - In a teapot or heat-resistant container, combine the dried hibiscus petals, lavender buds, chamomile flowers, and lemon balm leaves.

2. Infuse the Herbs:
   - Pour hot water over the herbs in the teapot. Cover and let it steep for about 10-15 minutes.

3. Strain the Elixir:
   - After steeping, strain the liquid through a fine mesh strainer or tea infuser into a clean mug or teacup.

4. Sweeten (Optional):
   - If desired, add 1-2 teaspoons of raw honey to the elixir and stir until dissolved. Adjust sweetness to your preference.

5. Sip and Enjoy:
   - Sip the elixir slowly about 30 minutes before bedtime to enjoy the calming and soothing properties of the herbs.

### Hibiscus Lavender Sleep Elixir Background:

- **Hibiscus:** Known for its bright and tangy flavor, hibiscus adds a vibrant touch to the elixir while contributing potential antioxidant benefits.

- **Lavender:** Renowned for its calming and relaxing properties, lavender is often used to promote a sense of tranquility and better sleep.

- **Chamomile:** A classic herb for relaxation, chamomile has mild sedative effects and may help ease stress and tension.

- **Lemon Balm:** With a gentle lemony flavor, lemon balm is known for its calming and mood-enhancing properties, contributing to the elixir's soothing effects.

Feel free to adjust the proportions based on your taste preferences, and enjoy this aromatic and calming sleep elixir as part of your bedtime routine. As always, if you have any specific health concerns or are taking medications, it's advisable to consult with a healthcare professional before introducing new herbs into your routine.

## Hibiscus Digestive Tincture with Traditional Chinese Medicine (TCM) Ingredients

This Hibiscus Digestive Tincture, enriched with TCM ingredients, aims to balance the body's energies and support overall digestive health. As always, consult with a healthcare professional, especially if you have specific health concerns or are taking medications.

### Ingredients:

- 2 tablespoons dried hibiscus petals
- 1 tablespoon dried ginger slices
- 1 tablespoon dried orange peel
- 1 teaspoon fennel seeds
- 1 teaspoon dried mint leaves
- 1 teaspoon dried licorice root
- 1 cup high-proof alcohol (e.g., vodka or brandy)

### Instructions:

1. Prepare the Herbs:
   - In a clean glass jar with a tight-fitting lid, combine the dried hibiscus petals, dried ginger slices, dried orange peel, fennel seeds, dried mint leaves, and dried licorice root.

2. Add Alcohol:
   - Pour the high-proof alcohol over the herbs, ensuring they are fully submerged. The alcohol acts as a solvent to extract the active compounds.

3. Maceration:
   - Seal the jar tightly and place it in a cool, dark place for 4-6 weeks. Shake the jar gently every few days to facilitate the maceration process.

4. Strain the Tincture:
   - After the maceration period, strain the liquid through a fine mesh strainer or cheesecloth into a clean glass container. Squeeze the herbs to extract any remaining liquid.

5. Bottle and Store:
   - Transfer the strained tincture into dark glass bottles with dropper lids. Store the bottles in a cool, dark place.

6. Usage:
   - Start with a small dose, such as 1/2 to 1 dropperful, before or after meals to aid in digestion. Adjust the dosage as needed.

### TCM Ingredients and Their Roles:

- **Hibiscus Petals (Hibiscus sabdariffa):**
  - Cooling nature, promotes fluid balance, and may help soothe the digestive system.

- **Ginger (Zingiber officinale):**
  - Warm nature, stimulates digestion, and helps alleviate nausea and bloating.

- **Orange Peel (Citrus sinensis):**
  - Aids in regulating Qi (vital energy), promotes digestion, and adds a citrusy flavor.

- **Fennel Seeds (Foeniculum vulgare):**
  - Warm nature, harmonizes the stomach, and relieves bloating and indigestion.

- **Mint Leaves (Mentha spp.):**
  - Cooling nature, soothes the digestive tract, and adds a refreshing element.

- **Licorice Root (Glycyrrhiza glabra):**
  - Harmonizes the formula, enhances flavor, and has potential anti-inflammatory properties.

## Hibiscus Skin Radiance Elixir

This Hibiscus Skin Radiance Elixir, enhanced with unexpected ingredients, offers a delightful and nourishing experience for your skin. Enjoy it as a part of your self-care routine, and revel in the natural beauty benefits of these thoughtfully chosen botanicals.

**Ingredients:**

- 2 tablespoons dried hibiscus petals
- 1 tablespoon dried calendula flowers
- 1 tablespoon dried chamomile flowers
- 1 teaspoon dried rose petals (unexpected ingredient)
- 1 teaspoon dried goji berries (unexpected ingredient)
- 1 cup hot water
- 1-2 teaspoons raw honey (optional, for sweetness)

**Instructions:**

1. Prepare the Herbs:
   - In a teapot or heat-resistant container, combine the dried hibiscus petals, calendula flowers, chamomile flowers, dried rose petals, and dried goji berries.

2. Infuse the Herbs:
   - Pour hot water over the herbs in the teapot. Cover and let it steep for about 10-15 minutes.

3. Strain the Elixir:
   - After steeping, strain the liquid through a fine mesh strainer or tea infuser into a clean mug or teacup.

4. Sweeten (Optional):
   - If desired, add 1-2 teaspoons of raw honey to the elixir and stir until dissolved. Adjust sweetness to your preference.

5. Sip and Enjoy:
   - Sip the elixir slowly, allowing the vibrant blend of hibiscus, calendula, chamomile, rose petals, and goji berries to nourish your skin from within.

**Unexpected Ingredients and Their Benefits:**

- **Rose Petals:**
  - Rose petals contribute a delicate floral note and are rich in antioxidants. They may help soothe the skin, reduce redness, and provide a subtle aromatic essence.

- **Goji Berries:**
  - Goji berries are packed with vitamins and antioxidants. They add a sweet touch to the elixir and may contribute to skin health by providing essential nutrients.

**Skin Radiance Elixir Background:**

- **Hibiscus (Hibiscus sabdariffa):**
  - Known for its brightening properties, hibiscus may support a radiant complexion and is rich in antioxidants that promote skin health.

- **Calendula (Calendula officinalis):**
  - Calendula is celebrated for its skin-soothing properties. It may help calm irritation and support a healthy glow.

- **Chamomile (Matricaria chamomilla):**
  - Chamomile is renowned for its calming effects, making it ideal for promoting skin radiance and reducing redness.

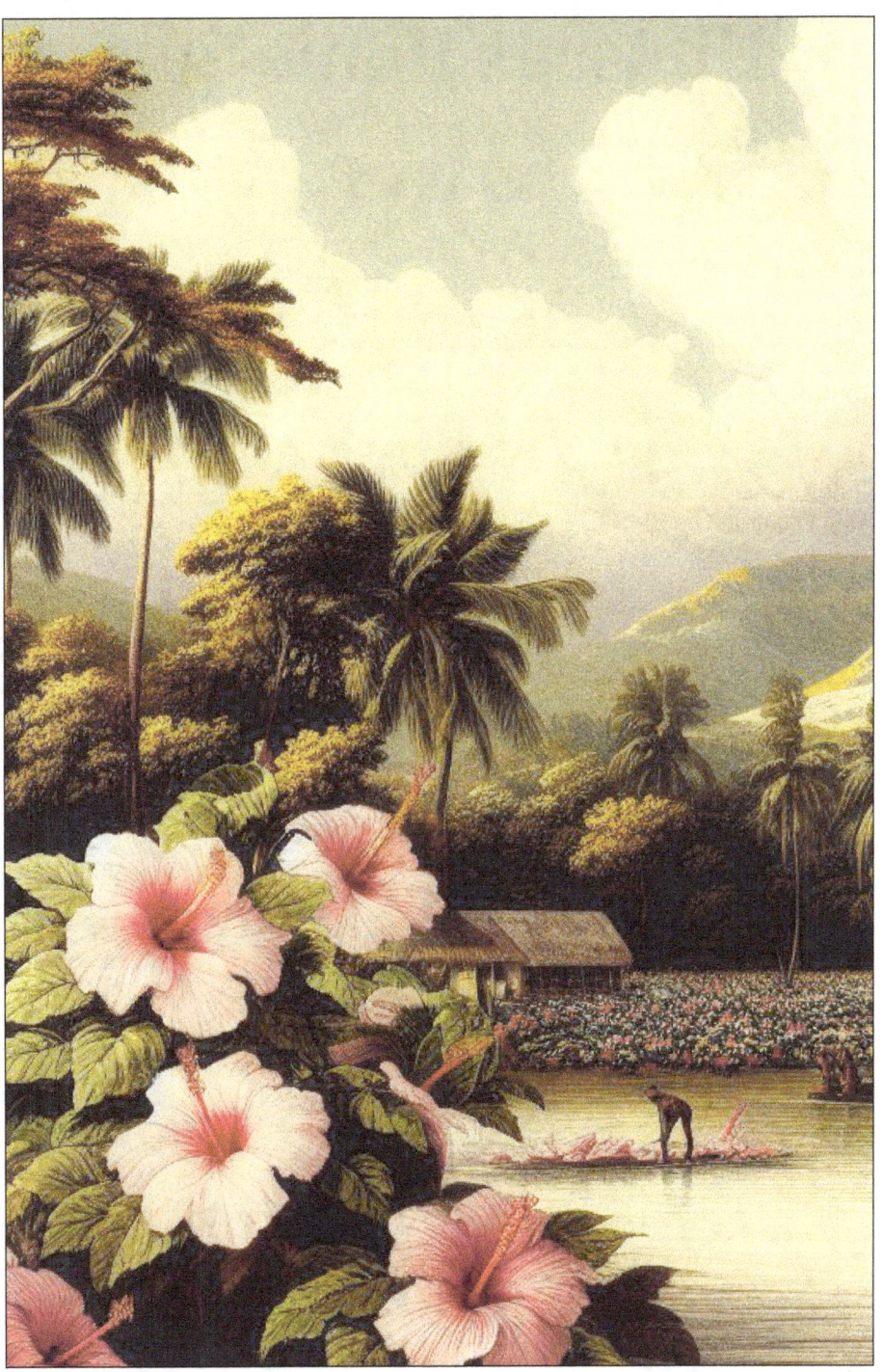

# Hibiscus Home Spa

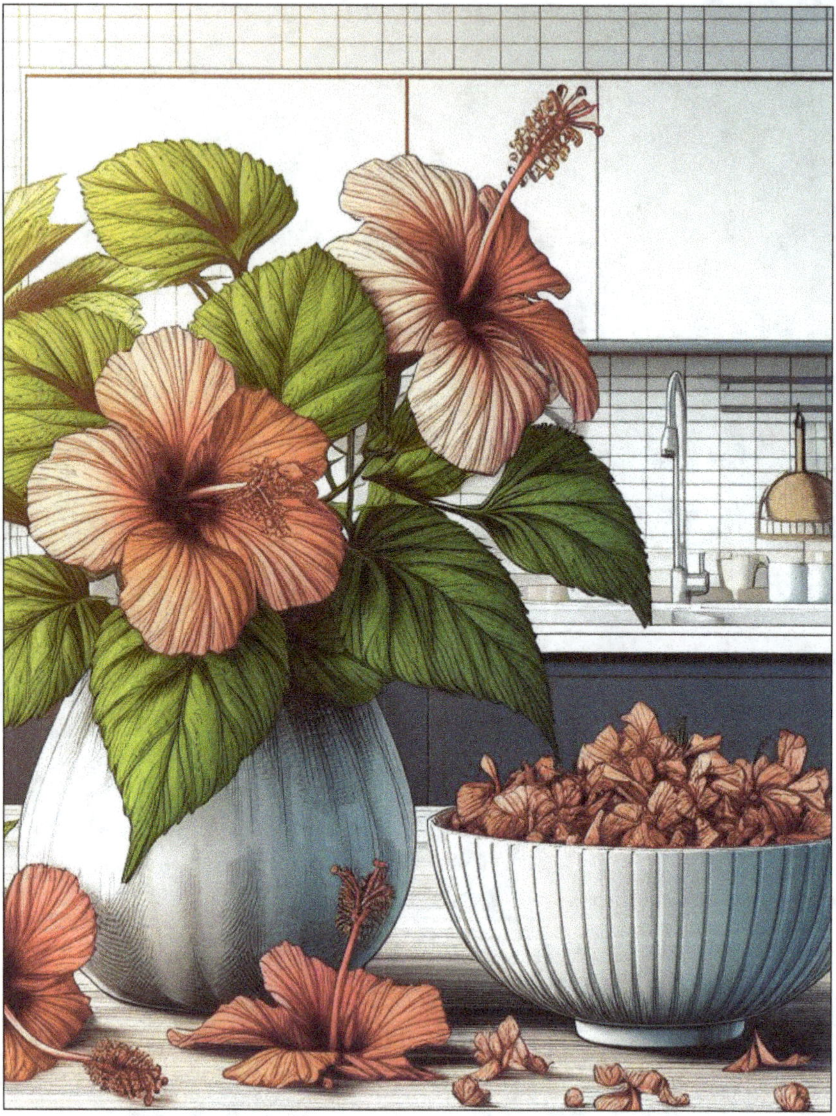

## Introduction to Creating Hibiscus-Based Home Spa Products:

Welcome to the world of DIY home spa products, where the beauty of nature meets the tranquility of self-care. In this journey, we'll explore the incredible potential of hibiscus – a vibrant and versatile botanical – as the cornerstone of our homemade spa recipes. Hibiscus, with its rich history and numerous skincare benefits, brings a touch of luxury and efficacy to each pampering session.

### Why Hibiscus?

**1. Radiant Skin Elixir:**
- Hibiscus is renowned for promoting radiant skin. Rich in antioxidants, it helps combat free radicals, reducing the signs of aging and leaving your skin with a youthful glow.

**2. Natural Exfoliation:**
- The natural acids present in hibiscus contribute to gentle exfoliation, removing dead skin cells and promoting a smoother complexion.

**3. Hydration Booster:**
- Hibiscus is a natural humectant, helping the skin retain moisture. This makes it an excellent ingredient for hydrating masks, scrubs, and treatments.

**4. Anti-Inflammatory Properties:**
- The anti-inflammatory and soothing properties of hibiscus make it ideal for calming irritated skin, reducing redness, and providing relief to sensitive areas.

**5. Hair Nourishment:**
- Beyond skincare, hibiscus nourishes and strengthens hair. It has been traditionally used to improve hair health, making it a valuable addition to hair masks and rinses.

**6. Aromatic Sensation:**
- The vibrant color and delightful fragrance of hibiscus petals add an aromatic dimension to your home spa experience, creating a sensory journey of relaxation.

**7. Versatility in Formulations:**
- Whether crafting facial masks, bath soaks, hair treatments, or teas, hibiscus seamlessly integrates into various formulations, offering a wide range of DIY spa possibilities.

### Our DIY Home Spa Journey:

As we embark on this journey, each recipe will showcase the multifaceted nature of hibiscus, coupled with carefully chosen ingredients to enhance your spa experience. From facial masks to body scrubs, hair treatments, and beyond, you'll discover the art of self-care using natural, accessible ingredients.

Prepare to indulge your senses, rejuvenate your skin, and create a spa retreat in the comfort of your own home, all with the vibrant and nurturing essence of hibiscus as our guide. Let the journey begin!

## Hibiscus and Green Tea Face Toner Ice Cubes

Hibiscus and green tea have been used for centuries in traditional medicine and skincare. Hibiscus is native to tropical regions and is often referred to as the "Botox plant" due to its skin-firming properties. Green tea has deep roots in Asian cultures, celebrated for its health benefits and skincare properties. Both ingredients have stood the test of time, recognized for their contributions to skincare and overall well-being.

**Ingredients:**

- Hibiscus tea (brewed and cooled)
- Green tea (brewed and cooled)
- Ice cube trays

Optional Add-ins:
- Aloe vera gel
- Cucumber juice
- Witch hazel
- Mint leaves (for a refreshing scent)

**Instructions:**

1. Brew the Teas:
   - Prepare hibiscus tea and green tea separately by steeping one hibiscus tea bag or a tablespoon of dried hibiscus petals and one green tea bag or a teaspoon of loose green tea leaves in hot water. Let them cool to room temperature.

2. Mixing the Teas:
   - In a bowl, mix equal parts of the cooled hibiscus tea and green tea. You can adjust the concentration based on your preference.

3. Optional Add-ins:
   - If desired, add a tablespoon of aloe vera gel for its soothing properties. You can also include a splash of cucumber juice for added freshness, a tablespoon of witch hazel for toning, or a few crushed mint leaves for a delightful scent.

4. Pour into Ice Cube Trays:
   - Pour the mixture into ice cube trays. This allows you to conveniently store and use the toner in individual portions.

5. Freeze:
   - Place the ice cube trays in the freezer and let the toner cubes freeze completely. This usually takes a few hours.

6. Usage:
   - Once frozen, take out one toner cube at a time and wrap it in a thin cloth or use it directly on your cleansed face. Gently rub the ice cube in circular motions, focusing on areas prone to redness or inflammation.

**Benefits:**
- Hibiscus: Rich in antioxidants, hibiscus helps purify the skin by fighting free radicals. It's known for its anti-aging properties, promoting a youthful complexion.
- Green Tea: Contains catechins that have anti-inflammatory and antioxidant properties. Green tea helps soothe the skin, reduce redness, and combat signs of aging.
- Aloe Vera: Provides hydration and has a cooling effect, perfect for soothing irritated or sun-exposed skin.
- Cucumber: Known for its refreshing properties, cucumber helps reduce puffiness and calms the skin.
- Witch Hazel: Acts as a natural astringent, tightening pores and reducing inflammation.

## Hibiscus and Honey Lip Balm

The hibiscus-infused oil contributes antioxidants, while beeswax forms a natural barrier to retain moisture. The addition of honey brings antibacterial properties, and a touch of essential oil enhances the balm with a delightful aroma and potential added benefits. Easy to make, this lip balm offers a soothing solution for dry or chapped lips, leaving them soft, moisturized, and subtly fragrant. Enjoy the natural goodness of hibiscus and honey in a convenient, homemade lip care essential.

### Ingredients:

- 2 tablespoons hibiscus-infused oil (hibiscus petals infused in a carrier oil like coconut oil or sweet almond oil)
- 1 tablespoon beeswax pellets or grated beeswax
- 1 teaspoon honey
- 5-7 drops of your preferred essential oil (e.g., lavender, vanilla, or peppermint)
- Lip balm containers or small jars

### Instructions:

1. Prepare Hibiscus-Infused Oil:
   - Place dried hibiscus petals in a jar and cover them with a carrier oil of your choice. Seal the jar and let it sit in a cool, dark place for at least two weeks. Strain the oil, and you now have hibiscus-infused oil.

2. Double Boiler Method:
   - In a heatproof container or the top part of a double boiler, combine the hibiscus-infused oil and beeswax pellets.

3. Melt the Ingredients:
   - Gently heat the mixture over low to medium heat until the beeswax completely melts. Stir occasionally to ensure even melting.

4. Add Honey:
   - Once the beeswax is melted, add the honey to the mixture. Stir well to combine. Honey adds moisturizing and antibacterial properties to the lip balm.

5. Essential Oil:
   - Add 5-7 drops of your preferred essential oil to the mixture. Essential oils not only contribute to the aroma but also provide additional benefits for the lips.

6. Pour into Containers:
   - Carefully pour the liquid lip balm into lip balm containers or small jars. Work quickly before the mixture solidifies.

7. Cool and Solidify:
   - Allow the lip balm to cool and solidify at room temperature. This may take a couple of hours.

8. Label and Store:
   - Once the lip balm has solidified, label the containers with the ingredients and date. Store them in a cool, dry place.

### Benefits:

- Hibiscus-Infused Oil: Rich in antioxidants, hibiscus helps nourish and protect the delicate skin on your lips.
- Beeswax: Provides a natural barrier that helps to seal in moisture and protect your lips from environmental factors.
- Honey: Acts as a humectant, attracting and retaining moisture. It also has antibacterial properties.
- Essential Oil: Adds a pleasant fragrance and may offer additional benefits, depending on the chosen oil.

### Usage:

- Apply the hibiscus and honey lip balm as needed to keep your lips moisturized and protected. Enjoy the natural benefits of the ingredients for soft and nourished lips.

## Hibiscus and Chamomile Eye Pillow

Drawing inspiration from ancient remedies and traditional medicine, this hibiscus and chamomile eye pillow transcends time, offering a natural solution for relieving eye strain, tension, and promoting a restful state of mind. The optional heating or chilling feature further elevates the experience, creating a personalized relaxation ritual that echoes the historical significance of these botanicals in holistic well-being practices. Immerse yourself in the gentle embrace of this eye pillow, where the past meets present in a restorative blend of nature's timeless gifts.

### Hibiscus:
Hibiscus has a rich history dating back centuries and has been cherished in various cultures for its diverse applications. Ancient Egyptians used hibiscus tea for its refreshing taste, while Ayurvedic medicine embraced its medicinal properties. In the Caribbean, hibiscus flowers were infused into skincare treatments due to their antioxidant content. The plant's vibrant petals have consistently found their way into traditional remedies, often symbolizing rejuvenation and well-being.

### Chamomile:
Chamomile, with its small, daisy-like flowers, boasts an extensive history as a therapeutic herb. Ancient Egyptians revered chamomile for its healing properties, incorporating it into medicinal infusions. The Greeks and Romans valued chamomile for its calming effects and digestive benefits. Additionally, in medieval Europe, chamomile was a staple in traditional folk medicine, renowned for its ability to ease stress and induce relaxation.

**Ingredients:**
- 1 cup dried hibiscus petals
- 1 cup dried chamomile flowers
- 1 cup flaxseeds or rice
- 1 tablespoon lavender buds (optional)
- 10-15 drops chamomile essential oil (optional)
- Soft, breathable fabric
- Ribbon or elastic band

**Instructions:**

1. Blend Herbs:
   - Mix hibiscus petals, chamomile flowers, flaxseeds/rice, and lavender buds (if using).

2. Add Essential Oil (Optional):
   - Include chamomile essential oil for a soothing scent.

3. Sew Pillow:
   - Cut and sew fabric into a pouch, leaving one side open.

4. Fill and Seal:
   - Fill pouch with the herbal blend, then securely stitch the open side.

5. Attach Band:
   - Add a ribbon or elastic band for easy securing.

6. Heat or Chill (Optional):
   - Warm in the microwave or chill in the fridge for added relaxation.

# Hibiscus and Peppermint Cooling Face Gel

This hibiscus and peppermint cooling face gel offers a natural and invigorating solution for a revitalized and refreshed complexion.

## Ingredients:

- 1 cup hibiscus tea (cooled)
- 2 tablespoons aloe vera gel
- 1/2 teaspoon peppermint essential oil
- 1-2 drops vitamin E oil (optional)
- 1 teaspoon glycerin (optional for added moisture)
- Mixing bowl
- Whisk or spoon
- Airtight container

## Instructions:

1. Brew Hibiscus Tea:
   - Steep hibiscus petals in hot water to create a concentrated tea. Allow it to cool to room temperature.

2. Prepare Aloe Vera Gel:
   - Ensure your aloe vera gel is pure and free from additives. Fresh aloe vera gel directly from the plant is ideal, but store-bought versions work as well.

3. Mixing the Gel:
   - In a mixing bowl, combine 1 cup of cooled hibiscus tea with 2 tablespoons of aloe vera gel. Stir well to ensure a smooth consistency.

4. Add Peppermint Essential Oil:
   - Incorporate 1/2 teaspoon of peppermint essential oil into the mixture. Adjust the quantity based on your preference, keeping in mind that peppermint provides a cooling sensation.

5. Optional Add-ins:
   - For added benefits, consider adding 1-2 drops of vitamin E oil for skin nourishment. Glycerin can be included for extra moisture, especially if you have dry skin. Mix thoroughly.

6. Transfer to Container:
   - Pour the mixture into a clean, airtight container. Choose a container that is easy to scoop the gel from and keeps the product sealed to maintain freshness.

7. Refrigerate (Optional):
   - For an enhanced cooling effect, you can refrigerate the gel before use. This is particularly refreshing during warm weather.

8. Usage:
   - Apply a small amount of the hibiscus and peppermint cooling face gel onto your clean face. Gently massage into your skin using upward circular motions. Use it as part of your skincare routine, particularly after cleansing.

## Benefits:

**Hibiscus:**
   - Rich in antioxidants, hibiscus helps soothe and refresh the skin. It also supports a radiant complexion.

**Aloe Vera Gel:**
   - Provides hydration and has a soothing effect on the skin. Aloe vera is known for its calming properties.

**Peppermint Essential Oil:**
   - Imparts a cooling sensation to the skin, making it perfect for a refreshing face gel. Peppermint oil can also help alleviate skin irritation.

**Vitamin E Oil (Optional):**
   - Adds moisture and nourishment, supporting the overall health of the skin.

**Glycerin (Optional):**
   - Enhances the moisturizing properties of the gel, particularly beneficial for individuals with dry skin.

## Hibiscus and Matcha Green Tea Face Scrub

This hibiscus and matcha green tea face scrub offers a rejuvenating and natural way to exfoliate your skin, leaving it refreshed and glowing.

### Ingredients:

- 1 tablespoon hibiscus powder
- 1 tablespoon matcha green tea powder
- 2 tablespoons sugar (white or brown)
- 2 tablespoons coconut oil (or any carrier oil of your choice)
- 1-2 drops of your favorite essential oil (optional, for fragrance)
- Mixing bowl
- Spoon
- Airtight container

### Instructions:

1. Combine Dry Ingredients:
   - In a mixing bowl, blend 1 tablespoon of hibiscus powder and 1 tablespoon of matcha green tea powder. These powders serve as the exfoliating and antioxidant-rich base for your scrub.

2. Add Sugar:
   - Incorporate 2 tablespoons of sugar into the dry ingredients. Sugar acts as an excellent natural exfoliant, helping to remove dead skin cells.

3. Introduce Carrier Oil:
   - Pour 2 tablespoons of coconut oil (or your chosen carrier oil) into the mixture. The oil provides moisture and helps bind the scrub together. Adjust the oil quantity based on your desired consistency.

4. Optional Fragrance:
   - If you desire a pleasant fragrance, add 1-2 drops of your favorite essential oil into the mix. Consider oils like lavender, chamomile, or vanilla for a soothing aroma.

5. Mix Thoroughly:
   - Use a spoon to thoroughly mix all the ingredients until you achieve a consistent, grainy texture. Ensure that the oil is evenly distributed.

6. Test and Adjust:
   - Test a small amount of the scrub on your hand. If you prefer a smoother texture, you can add more oil. For a coarser scrub, add more sugar.

7. Transfer to Container:
   - Once satisfied with the consistency, transfer the hibiscus and matcha green tea face scrub into an airtight container. This preserves the freshness of the ingredients.

8. Usage:
   - Apply a small amount of the scrub to dampened skin. Gently massage in circular motions, focusing on areas that may need extra exfoliation. Rinse thoroughly with warm water.

### Benefits:

**Hibiscus:**
- Packed with antioxidants, hibiscus promotes skin renewal and helps maintain a youthful glow. It also has natural exfoliating properties.

**Matcha Green Tea:**
- Known for its anti-inflammatory properties, matcha green tea soothes the skin and provides antioxidants to combat free radicals.

**Sugar:**
- Acts as a physical exfoliant, helping to remove dead skin cells and promote a smoother complexion.

**Coconut Oil:**
- Provides moisture and nourishment to the skin, leaving it soft and supple.

## Hibiscus and Ylang-Ylang Relaxing Pillow Mist

This DIY hibiscus and ylang-ylang relaxing pillow mist offers a simple yet effective way to enhance your sleep environment, transforming your bedtime routine into a calming and aromatic experience.

### Ingredients:

- 1 cup hibiscus tea (cooled)
- 10-15 drops ylang-ylang essential oil
- 1 tablespoon witch hazel
- Distilled water
- Spray bottle

### Instructions:

1. Brew Hibiscus Tea:
   - Steep hibiscus petals in hot water to create a concentrated tea. Allow it to cool to room temperature, then strain to remove the petals.

2. Prepare the Mist Base:
   - In a mixing bowl, combine 1 cup of cooled hibiscus tea with 1 tablespoon of witch hazel. Witch hazel acts as a natural emulsifier and helps the mist disperse evenly.

3. Add Ylang-Ylang Essential Oil:
   - Introduce 10-15 drops of ylang-ylang essential oil to the hibiscus tea and witch hazel base. Adjust the number of drops based on your preference, considering ylang-ylang's potent floral aroma.

4. Mix Thoroughly:
   - Stir the mixture well to ensure the essential oil is evenly distributed. This forms the aromatic and calming base for your pillow mist.

5. Transfer to Spray Bottle:
   - Using a funnel, pour the hibiscus and ylang-ylang mist into a clean spray bottle. Leave some space at the top to allow for proper misting.

6. Dilute with Distilled Water:
   - Top off the spray bottle with distilled water, leaving about an inch of space from the top. This dilution ensures a gentle mist that won't leave your pillow overly damp.

7. Shake Well:
   - Shake the bottle well before each use to mix the ingredients and activate the soothing properties of hibiscus and ylang-ylang.

8. Usage:
   - Spritz the mist lightly onto your pillow and bedding before bedtime. Allow the calming fragrance to envelop your senses, promoting relaxation and a peaceful sleep.

### Benefits:

**Hibiscus:**
- The aroma of hibiscus promotes tranquility, while its antioxidant properties contribute to a calming atmosphere.

**Ylang-Ylang Essential Oil:**
- Known for its floral and sweet aroma, ylang-ylang is valued for its ability to alleviate stress, reduce anxiety, and induce a sense of relaxation.

**Witch Hazel:**
- Acts as a natural emulsifier, helping the essential oil and tea blend evenly with water.

**Distilled Water:**
- Provides a gentle dilution, ensuring a light mist that won't saturate your pillow.

## Hibiscus and Oatmeal Face Mask

This hibiscus and oatmeal face mask provides a nourishing and rejuvenating treat for your skin, combining the benefits of these natural ingredients for a spa-like experience at home.

### Ingredients:

- 2 tablespoons hibiscus powder
- 2 tablespoons finely ground oatmeal
- 1-2 tablespoons plain yogurt
- 1 teaspoon honey
- Mixing bowl
- Spoon
- Optional: Rosewater or water for consistency

### Instructions:

1. Prepare Hibiscus Powder:
   - If you don't have hibiscus powder, grind dried hibiscus petals into a fine powder using a blender or spice grinder.

2. Combine Dry Ingredients:
   - In a mixing bowl, combine 2 tablespoons of hibiscus powder with 2 tablespoons of finely ground oatmeal. Oatmeal serves as a gentle exfoliant and helps soothe the skin.

3. Add Wet Ingredients:
   - Introduce 1-2 tablespoons of plain yogurt to the dry mixture. Yogurt provides a creamy base and contains lactic acid, contributing to gentle exfoliation and skin brightening.

4. Incorporate Honey:
   - Add 1 teaspoon of honey to the mixture. Honey is a natural humectant, attracting and retaining moisture for soft and supple skin.

5. Optional: Adjust Consistency:
   - If the mask is too thick, you can add a small amount of rosewater or regular water to achieve your desired consistency. Mix until you have a smooth and spreadable paste.

6. Test Patch:
   - Before applying the mask to your face, do a patch test on a small area of your skin to ensure there is no irritation.

7. Application:
   - Using clean fingers or a brush, apply the hibiscus and oatmeal face mask evenly to your face, avoiding the eye area. Gently massage in circular motions for exfoliation.

8. Relax and Rinse:
   - Allow the mask to sit for 15-20 minutes. Relax and enjoy the soothing properties. Rinse off with lukewarm water, pat your face dry, and follow up with your favorite moisturizer.

### Benefits:

**Hibiscus:**
- Rich in antioxidants, hibiscus helps brighten the skin, reduce the appearance of fine lines, and promotes a youthful complexion.

**Oatmeal:**
- Acts as a gentle exfoliant, helping to remove dead skin cells and soothe irritated skin. Oatmeal is known for its calming properties.

**Yogurt:**
- Contains lactic acid, providing mild exfoliation and contributing to a more even skin tone. The probiotics in yogurt can also help nourish the skin.

**Honey:**
- Offers natural antibacterial properties and helps moisturize the skin, leaving it soft and hydrated.

## Hibiscus and Lemon Cuticle Oil

This DIY hibiscus and lemon cuticle oil is a luxurious and natural way to care for your nails and cuticles, leaving them looking and feeling revitalized.

### Ingredients:

- 2 tablespoons hibiscus-infused oil (hibiscus petals infused in a carrier oil like sweet almond oil or jojoba oil)
- 1 tablespoon olive oil (or another carrier oil of your choice)
- 10 drops lemon essential oil
- Vitamin E oil capsule (optional for added nourishment)
- Small glass dropper bottle

### Instructions:

1. Prepare Hibiscus-Infused Oil:
   - Infuse hibiscus petals in a carrier oil of your choice (such as sweet almond oil or jojoba oil). Place dried hibiscus petals in a jar, cover with the carrier oil, and let it sit in a cool, dark place for at least two weeks. Strain the oil to remove the petals.

2. Mix Carrier Oils:
   - In a small bowl, combine 2 tablespoons of hibiscus-infused oil with 1 tablespoon of olive oil. This blend provides a nourishing base for your cuticle oil.

3. Add Lemon Essential Oil:
   - Incorporate 10 drops of lemon essential oil into the mixture. Lemon oil adds a refreshing scent and has natural antiseptic properties.

4. Optional: Vitamin E Oil:
   - If you have a vitamin E oil capsule, puncture it and squeeze the oil into the mixture. Vitamin E is known for its skin-nourishing and antioxidant properties.

5. Stir Well:
   - Stir the ingredients well to ensure they are thoroughly combined.

6. Transfer to Dropper Bottle:
   - Using a small funnel, pour the hibiscus and lemon cuticle oil mixture into a glass dropper bottle. This makes application convenient and mess-free.

7. Shake Before Use:
   - Before each use, shake the bottle well to mix the oils.

8. Usage:
   - Apply a small amount of the cuticle oil to your nails and cuticles. Gently massage the oil into the skin, promoting circulation and providing nourishment. Use regularly for healthier-looking nails and cuticles.

### Benefits:

Hibiscus-Infused Oil:
   - Rich in antioxidants, hibiscus-infused oil helps promote healthy nails and cuticles. It also contributes to strengthening the nails.

Olive Oil:
   - Provides moisture to the cuticles, preventing dryness and promoting flexibility.

Lemon Essential Oil:
   - Offers a fresh and invigorating scent. Lemon oil also has natural antiseptic properties, helping to keep the cuticles clean.

Vitamin E Oil (Optional):
   - Supports overall nail health by providing nourishment and protecting against free radicals.

## Hibiscus Facial Steam

### History of Facial Steaming:

Facial steaming has deep historical roots in various cultures:

- **Ancient Rome:** Romans were known to use steam baths for both hygiene and relaxation.

- **Traditional Chinese Medicine:** Chinese medicine incorporates facial steaming to enhance blood circulation and promote skin health.

- **Ayurveda:** The ancient Indian practice of Ayurveda emphasizes steam treatments, known as "swedana," to purify the skin and balance doshas.

- **Native American Traditions:** Native American tribes utilized steam baths, often incorporating herbal infusions, for spiritual and physical purification.

Facial steaming is valued for its ability to open pores, enhance circulation, and promote relaxation. The addition of hibiscus brings antioxidant and skin-soothing benefits to this time-honored practice.

### Ingredients:

- 2 tablespoons dried hibiscus petals
- 4 cups hot water
- Optional: Essential oils (lavender, chamomile) for added aromatherapy
- Large heatproof bowl
- Towel

### Instructions:

1. Prepare Hibiscus Petals:
   - Place 2 tablespoons of dried hibiscus petals in a large heatproof bowl.

2. Boil Water:
   - Boil 4 cups of water and pour it over the hibiscus petals in the bowl.

3. Add Optional Essential Oils:
   - Optionally, add a few drops of essential oils like lavender or chamomile for added relaxation and aromatherapy benefits.

4. Cover and Steep:
   - Cover your head with a towel, creating a tent over the bowl. Ensure the towel drapes over the sides to trap the steam.

5. Steam Your Face:
   - Position your face over the bowl, keeping a comfortable distance to avoid burns. Close your eyes and breathe deeply, allowing the steam to open your pores.

6. Steam for 10-15 Minutes:
   - Enjoy the facial steam for 10-15 minutes, allowing the hibiscus-infused steam to work its magic on your skin.

7. Follow with Skincare Routine:
   - After steaming, follow up with your regular skincare routine. The open pores are more receptive to skincare products.

### Variations:

1. **Herbal Blend:**
   - Combine hibiscus with other herbs like chamomile, lavender, or rose petals for a diverse herbal steam.

2. **Citrus Infusion:**
   - Add a few citrus peels (orange or lemon) for a refreshing twist and additional skin-brightening benefits.

3. **Tea Blend:**
   - Mix hibiscus petals with green tea or chamomile tea for a soothing and antioxidant-rich facial steam.

4. **Eucalyptus Invigoration:**
   - Add a few drops of eucalyptus essential oil for a refreshing and invigorating facial steam, especially beneficial for congested skin.

# Hibiscus and Green Clay Face Pack

This hibiscus and green clay face pack provides a deep-cleansing and revitalizing experience for your skin, leaving it refreshed and rejuvenated.

### Ingredients:

- 1 tablespoon hibiscus powder
- 1 tablespoon green clay
- 2 tablespoons water (adjust as needed)
- 1 teaspoon honey
- Optional: 1-2 drops of essential oil (lavender, tea tree, or chamomile)
- Mixing bowl
- Spoon

### Instructions:

1. Combine Dry Ingredients:
   - In a mixing bowl, combine 1 tablespoon of hibiscus powder with 1 tablespoon of green clay. These ingredients work together to cleanse and revitalize the skin.

2. Add Water:
   - Gradually add water to the dry mixture, stirring continuously until you achieve a smooth and spreadable consistency. Adjust the amount of water as needed.

3. Incorporate Honey:
   - Mix in 1 teaspoon of honey. Honey adds moisture and has natural antibacterial properties, benefiting the skin.

4. Optional: Essential Oil:
   - If desired, add 1-2 drops of essential oil for a pleasant fragrance and potential additional skincare benefits. Essential oils like lavender, tea tree, or chamomile are good options.

5. Stir Well:
   - Ensure all ingredients are thoroughly mixed, forming a uniform paste.

6. Test Patch:
   - Before applying the face pack to your entire face, do a patch test on a small area of your skin to ensure there is no irritation.

7. Application:
   - Using clean fingers or a brush, apply the hibiscus and green clay face pack evenly to your face, avoiding the eye and lip area.

8. Relax and Rinse:
   - Allow the face pack to dry for about 15-20 minutes. Relax during this time, and once the pack has hardened, rinse it off with warm water. Gently pat your face dry.

### Benefits:

**Hibiscus:**
 - Rich in antioxidants, hibiscus promotes skin renewal, helps tighten pores, and adds a natural glow.

**Green Clay:**
 - Known for its detoxifying properties, green clay absorbs excess oil and impurities, leaving the skin refreshed.

**Honey:**
 - Offers antibacterial properties and adds moisture, making the skin soft and supple.

**Essential Oils (Optional):**
 - Lavender, tea tree, or chamomile essential oils contribute fragrance and potential skincare benefits, such as calming or anti-inflammatory effects.

This hibiscus and green clay face pack provides a deep-cleansing and revitalizing experience for your skin, leaving it refreshed and rejuvenated.

## Hibiscus and Rose Petal Bath Salts

Ingredients:

- 1 cup Epsom salts
- 1/4 cup dried hibiscus petals
- 1/4 cup dried rose petals
- 1/4 cup sea salt
- 1 tablespoon hibiscus powder
- 1 tablespoon dried rosehip (optional)
- 10-15 drops rose essential oil
- Mixing bowl
- Airtight container or glass jar

Instructions:

1. Prepare Dried Petals:
   - Ensure the hibiscus and rose petals are thoroughly dried. You can air-dry them or use a dehydrator.

2. Crush Petals:
   - In a mixing bowl, crush the dried hibiscus and rose petals gently with your hands to release their fragrance.

3. Combine Salts:
   - Add 1 cup of Epsom salts and 1/4 cup of sea salt to the crushed petals in the bowl.

4. Add Hibiscus Powder and Rosehip (Optional):
   - Include 1 tablespoon of hibiscus powder and, if desired, 1 tablespoon of dried rosehip for additional benefits. Rosehip is rich in vitamins and antioxidants.

5. Introduce Rose Essential Oil:
   - Add 10-15 drops of rose essential oil to the mixture. Adjust the quantity based on your preference for scent strength.

6. Mix Thoroughly:
   - Stir all the ingredients together until well combined. Ensure that the essential oil is evenly distributed.

7. Transfer to Container:
   - Carefully transfer the hibiscus and rose petal bath salts into an airtight container or glass jar.

8. Seal and Store:
   - Seal the container or jar tightly to preserve the freshness of the bath salts. Store in a cool, dry place.

Usage:

1. Bathing Ritual:
   - Add a generous handful of the hibiscus and rose petal bath salts to warm running bathwater.

2. Relax and Soak:
   - Immerse yourself in the bath, allowing the salts to dissolve and the floral fragrance to envelop you. Relax and soak for at least 20 minutes.

3. Rinse:
   - After soaking, rinse off in a warm shower to remove any residual salts from your skin.

Benefits:

Hibiscus:
   - Rich in antioxidants, hibiscus promotes skin health and adds a vibrant color to the bath.

Rose Petals:
   - Contributes a delicate fragrance and offers potential skin-soothing benefits.

Epsom Salts:
   - Contains magnesium, which can help relax muscles and promote a sense of calm.

Sea Salt:
   - Adds minerals to the bath and may help with detoxification.

Rose Essential Oil:
   - Imparts a luxurious and calming scent, promoting relaxation.

## Hibiscus and Honey Face Wash

### Ingredients:

- 1 tablespoon hibiscus powder
- 1 tablespoon raw honey
- 1 teaspoon aloe vera gel
- 1 teaspoon jojoba oil (or your preferred carrier oil)
- 2-3 drops tea tree essential oil (optional, for added antibacterial properties)
- Mixing bowl
- Spoon
- Airtight container

### Instructions:

1. Prepare Hibiscus Powder:
   - If you don't have hibiscus powder, grind dried hibiscus petals into a fine powder using a blender or spice grinder.

2. Mix Dry Ingredients:
   - In a mixing bowl, combine 1 tablespoon hibiscus powder with 1 tablespoon raw honey. Mix well to form a smooth paste.

3. Add Aloe Vera Gel:
   - Incorporate 1 teaspoon of aloe vera gel into the mixture. Aloe vera is soothing and helps balance the skin's moisture.

4. Introduce Carrier Oil:
   - Add 1 teaspoon of jojoba oil (or your preferred carrier oil). Jojoba oil is known for its moisturizing properties and similarity to the skin's natural oils.

5. Optional: Tea Tree Essential Oil:
   - If desired, add 2-3 drops of tea tree essential oil for its antibacterial and acne-fighting properties.

6. Stir Well:
   - Mix all the ingredients thoroughly until you achieve a well-blended consistency.

7. Transfer to Container:
   - Carefully transfer the hibiscus and honey face wash into an airtight container for storage.

### Usage:

1. Apply to Dampened Skin:
   - Wet your face with warm water and apply a small amount of the face wash to your dampened skin.

2. Gentle Massage:
   - Gently massage the face wash onto your skin in circular motions, avoiding the eye area.

3. Rinse Thoroughly:
   - Rinse your face thoroughly with lukewarm water, ensuring all the face wash is removed.

4. Pat Dry:
   - Pat your face dry with a clean towel and follow up with your favorite moisturizer.

### Benefits:

Hibiscus:
- Rich in antioxidants, hibiscus helps promote a radiant complexion and may aid in skin rejuvenation.

Honey:
- Provides natural antibacterial properties, helps moisturize the skin, and contributes to a healthy glow.

Aloe Vera Gel:
- Soothes and hydrates the skin, providing relief from irritation and redness.

Jojoba Oil:
- Mimics the skin's natural oils, offering hydration without clogging pores.

Tea Tree Essential Oil (Optional):
- Adds antibacterial properties, making it suitable for acne-prone skin.

## Hibiscus and Aloe Vera Cooling Gel

This DIY hibiscus and aloe vera cooling gel is a versatile and soothing solution for various skin needs, especially beneficial for calming and refreshing the skin after exposure to the sun or during hot weather.

Ingredients:

- 2 tablespoons hibiscus tea (cooled)
- 2 tablespoons aloe vera gel
- 1 teaspoon vegetable glycerin (optional, for added moisture)
- 2-3 drops peppermint essential oil (optional, for a cooling sensation)
- Mixing bowl
- Spoon
- Airtight container

Instructions:

1. Prepare Hibiscus Tea:
   - Steep hibiscus petals in hot water to create a hibiscus tea. Allow it to cool completely.

2. Combine Ingredients:
   - In a mixing bowl, blend 2 tablespoons of cooled hibiscus tea with 2 tablespoons of aloe vera gel.

3. Add Vegetable Glycerin (Optional):
   - If you desire extra moisture, include 1 teaspoon of vegetable glycerin and mix well.

4. Optional Peppermint Essential Oil:
   - For a cooling effect, add 2-3 drops of peppermint essential oil. Mix thoroughly.

5. Stir Well:
   - Ensure all ingredients are well combined to create a smooth gel consistency.

6. Transfer to Container:
   - Place the hibiscus and aloe vera cooling gel into an airtight container for storage.

Usage:

1. Apply to Sunburned or Irritated Skin:

The hibiscus and aloe vera cooling gel can help sunburnt skin by:

A. Hibiscus:
- Provides anti-inflammatory properties.
- Offers a mild cooling sensation.

B. Aloe Vera Gel:
- Soothes and cools the skin.
- Hydrates and prevents dryness.

C. Optional Ingredients:
- Vegetable glycerin adds extra moisture.
- Peppermint essential oil provides a cooling sensation.

How to Use:
- Gently apply to sunburnt areas for relief.
- Reapply as needed.
- Refrigerate for an added cooling effect.

While the gel offers relief, practicing sun protection is essential to prevent sunburn.

2. Soothing Facial Gel:
   - Apply a small amount to your face for a soothing and hydrating experience.

3. Refresh Your Body:
   - Apply to pulse points for a refreshing sensation on a hot day. A pulse point is a location on the body where the heartbeat can be easily felt due to arteries being close to the skin's surface. Common pulse points include the wrist, neck, temple, inside of the elbow, groin, and behind the knee. In skincare and aromatherapy, pulse points are areas where products are applied for enhanced absorption and diffusion.

# Hibiscus and Red Wine Anti-Aging Serum

This DIY hibiscus and red wine anti-aging serum provides a natural and luxurious addition to your skincare routine, aiming to nourish and revitalize the skin.

### Ingredients:

- 2 tablespoons dried hibiscus petals
- 1/4 cup red wine
- 1 teaspoon vitamin C serum
- 1 teaspoon rosehip oil
- Glass jar with lid
- Strainer or cheesecloth

### Instructions:

1. Prepare Dried Hibiscus Petals:
   - Ensure the hibiscus petals are thoroughly dried. You can air-dry them or use a dehydrator.

2. Combine Ingredients in Glass Jar:
   - In a glass jar, combine 2 tablespoons of dried hibiscus petals with 1/4 cup of red wine.

3. Add Vitamin C Serum:
   - Incorporate 1 teaspoon of vitamin C serum into the mixture. Vitamin C is known for its antioxidant properties, which can help promote collagen production.

4. Introduce Rosehip Oil:
   - Add 1 teaspoon of rosehip oil to the jar. Rosehip oil is rich in vitamins and essential fatty acids, contributing to skin hydration and elasticity.

5. Infuse for Several Weeks:
   - Seal the jar tightly and place it in a cool, dark place to infuse for several weeks. Shake the jar gently every few days to help extract the beneficial properties.

6. Strain the Mixture:
   - After the infusion period, strain the mixture using a fine mesh strainer or cheesecloth to separate the liquid from the hibiscus petals.

7. Transfer to a Dropper Bottle:
   - Pour the strained liquid into a dark glass dropper bottle for easy application and to preserve the serum.

### Usage:

1. Apply to Clean Skin:
   - Use the serum on clean, dry skin. You can apply it in the morning or evening.

2. Gently Massage:
   - Take a few drops of the serum and gently massage it onto your face and neck using upward motions.

3. Follow with Moisturizer:
   - Allow the serum to absorb into your skin and follow up with your favorite moisturizer.

### Benefits:

**Hibiscus:**
- Packed with antioxidants, hibiscus may help reduce the appearance of fine lines and wrinkles.

**Red Wine:**
- Red wine is a notable source of resveratrol, a polyphenol with potent antioxidant properties. Antioxidants help neutralize free radicals, protecting the skin from oxidative stress and damage caused by environmental factors like UV radiation and pollution.

**Vitamin C:**
- Promotes collagen synthesis and brightens the skin.

**Rosehip Oil:**
- Hydrates the skin and supports elasticity.

## Hibiscus and Turmeric Brightening Face Elixir

This DIY hibiscus and turmeric brightening face elixir aims to enhance your skin's radiance and promote an even complexion when used consistently as part of your nighttime skincare routine.

### Ingredients:

- 1 tablespoon hibiscus extract (prepared by steeping dried hibiscus petals in hot water)
- 1/2 teaspoon turmeric powder
- 1/2 teaspoon licorice root extract
- 2 tablespoons aloe vera gel
- Dark glass dropper bottle
- Mixing bowl
- Spoon

### Instructions:

1. Prepare Hibiscus Extract:
   - Steep dried hibiscus petals in hot water to create hibiscus extract. Allow it to cool before using.

2. Combine Ingredients:
   - In a mixing bowl, blend 1 tablespoon of hibiscus extract with 1/2 teaspoon of turmeric powder.

3. Add Licorice Root Extract:
   - Incorporate 1/2 teaspoon of licorice root extract into the mixture. Licorice root is known for its skin-brightening properties.

4. Introduce Aloe Vera Gel:
   - Add 2 tablespoons of aloe vera gel to the bowl. Aloe vera soothes the skin and provides additional hydration.

5. Mix Thoroughly:
   - Stir all the ingredients together until you achieve a smooth and well-blended consistency.

6. Transfer to Dropper Bottle:
   - Carefully pour the elixir into a dark glass dropper bottle. The dark glass helps protect the formulation from light, preserving its efficacy.

### Usage:

1. Apply Nightly:
   - Use the brightening elixir nightly as part of your skincare routine.

2. Cleanse Your Face:
   - Start with a clean, dry face before applying the elixir.

3. Use Dropper for Application:
   - With the dropper, dispense a few drops of the elixir onto your fingertips.

4. Gently Massage:
   - Gently massage the elixir onto your face and neck using upward motions.

5. Allow Absorption:
   - Allow the elixir to absorb into your skin. Follow up with your regular moisturizer if needed.

### Benefits:

**Hibiscus:**
- Rich in AHAs (alpha hydroxy acids) that promote exfoliation, revealing a brighter complexion.
- Contains antioxidants that may help with anti-aging.

**Turmeric:**
- Known for its anti-inflammatory and skin-brightening properties.

**Licorice Root Extract:**
- Offers skin-brightening effects and helps even out skin tone.

**Aloe Vera Gel:**
- Soothes and hydrates the skin, providing a calming effect.

# Hibiscus and Kakadu Plum Dark Spot Corrector

This DIY hibiscus and Kakadu plum dark spot corrector aims to address dark spots and promote a more even skin tone when used consistently as part of your skincare routine.

## Ingredients:

- 1 tablespoon hibiscus powder
- 1/2 teaspoon Kakadu plum extract
- 1/2 teaspoon bearberry extract
- A few drops of carrot seed oil
- Small bowl for mixing
- Spoon for stirring
- Dark glass jar or container

## Instructions:

1. Combine Hibiscus Powder and Extracts:
   - In a small bowl, mix 1 tablespoon of hibiscus powder with 1/2 teaspoon each of Kakadu plum extract and bearberry extract.

2. Add Carrot Seed Oil:
   - Incorporate a few drops of carrot seed oil into the mixture. Carrot seed oil is known for its skin-brightening and rejuvenating properties.

3. Stir Well:
   - Stir the ingredients thoroughly until you achieve a smooth and well-blended consistency.

4. Transfer to a Dark Glass Jar:
   - Carefully transfer the dark spot corrector into a dark glass jar or container. Dark glass helps protect the formulation from light, preserving its efficacy.

## Usage:

1. Apply on Targeted Areas:
   - Use the dark spot corrector on targeted areas where you have dark spots or hyperpigmentation.

2. Cleanse Your Face:
   - Begin with a clean, dry face before applying the corrector.

3. Use a Small Amount:
   - Take a small amount of the corrector on your fingertips.

4. Gently Massage:
   - Gently massage the corrector onto the targeted areas using circular motions.

5. Allow Absorption:
   - Allow the corrector to absorb into your skin.

6. Use Twice Daily:
   - For best results, use the corrector twice daily as part of your skincare routine.

## Benefits:

**Hibiscus:**
- Contains AHAs that may help exfoliate and brighten the skin.
- Rich in antioxidants that can contribute to skin health.

**Kakadu Plum Extract:**
- High in vitamin C, which supports collagen production and brightens the skin.

**Bearberry Extract:**
- Known for its skin-brightening properties and potential to reduce hyperpigmentation.

**Carrot Seed Oil:**
- Contains antioxidants and vitamins that may help with skin rejuvenation and even tone.

## Volcanic Ash and Hibiscus Facial Mask

The Volcanic Ash and Hibiscus Facial Mask is a potent skincare concoction that combines the detoxifying properties of volcanic ash with the nourishing and brightening benefits of hibiscus. This mask is designed to provide a spa-like experience in the comfort of your home, offering a range of benefits for your skin.

**Volcanic Ash Overview:**

Volcanic ash offers several benefits for skincare due to its unique composition and properties. Here are some of the key benefits:

**1. Exfoliation:** Volcanic ash contains fine particles that act as a natural exfoliant. When used in skincare products, it helps remove dead skin cells, unclog pores, and promote smoother skin texture.

**2. Detoxification:** The absorptive properties of volcanic ash make it effective in drawing out impurities, excess oil, and toxins from the skin. This detoxifying action can contribute to clearer and healthier-looking skin.

**3. Oil Control:** Volcanic ash has oil-absorbing qualities, making it beneficial for individuals with oily or combination skin. It helps to control excess oil production, reducing shine and minimizing the appearance of pores.

**4. Anti-Inflammatory:** The minerals found in volcanic ash, such as magnesium and zinc, have anti-inflammatory properties. These properties can help soothe irritated skin and reduce redness.

**5. Anti-Bacterial:** Volcanic ash possesses natural antibacterial properties, making it effective in combatting acne and preventing bacterial infections on the skin.

**6. Mineral Enrichment:** Volcanic ash is rich in minerals like silica, which is essential for maintaining the skin's elasticity and hydration. These minerals contribute to a healthier skin barrier.

**7. Improved Circulation:** When used in skincare treatments, volcanic ash can stimulate blood circulation. Improved blood flow helps deliver nutrients to skin cells and promotes a healthy complexion.

**8. Anti-Aging:** The exfoliating and rejuvenating effects of volcanic ash contribute to its anti-aging benefits. Regular use can help reduce the appearance of fine lines and wrinkles, promoting a more youthful-looking complexion.

**9. Soothing Properties:** Despite its abrasive nature, volcanic ash can have a soothing effect on the skin. It can help calm irritation and provide relief to sensitive skin when used in appropriate formulations.

**10. Environmental Protection:** Volcanic ash is often used in skincare products designed for environmental protection. It can help shield the skin from environmental pollutants and free radicals, which can contribute to premature aging.

It's important to note that while volcanic ash can offer benefits, individual skin reactions may vary. It's advisable to perform a patch test before using products containing volcanic ash, especially for those with sensitive skin. Additionally, incorporating volcanic ash into a balanced skincare routine, along with other beneficial ingredients, can enhance its effectiveness.

The combination of volcanic ash and hibiscus provides a powerful anti-aging effect, targeting fine lines, wrinkles, and signs of premature aging.

## Ingredients:

- 2 tablespoons volcanic ash powder
- 1 tablespoon dried hibiscus powder
- 1 tablespoon aloe vera gel
- 1 teaspoon raw honey
- 1-2 drops tea tree essential oil (optional, for added skin purification)
- Water (as needed)

## Instructions:

1. Combine Dry Ingredients:
   - In a small bowl, mix the volcanic ash powder and dried hibiscus powder together until well combined.

2. Add Wet Ingredients:
   - Add the aloe vera gel, raw honey, and tea tree essential oil (if using) to the dry ingredients.

3. Mix into a Paste:
   - Gradually add water, a little at a time, and stir until you achieve a smooth paste-like consistency. Ensure there are no lumps.

4. Application:
   - Cleanse your face thoroughly before applying the mask. Using clean fingers or a mask applicator, spread the mixture evenly over your face, avoiding the eye area.

5. Relax and Let it Dry:
   - Allow the mask to dry for about 15-20 minutes. As it dries, you may feel a tightening sensation.

6. Rinse Off:
   - Once the mask is dry, dampen your face with water and gently massage the mask using circular motions. Rinse thoroughly with lukewarm water.

7. Follow with Moisturizer:
   - Pat your face dry and follow up with your favorite moisturizer to keep your skin hydrated.

## Benefits of Ingredients:

- Volcanic Ash: see above

- Hibiscus Powder:
  - Hibiscus is rich in antioxidants and has exfoliating properties. It may help promote a smoother complexion and even out skin tone.

- Aloe Vera Gel:
  - Aloe vera is soothing and hydrating. It helps calm irritated skin and provides a refreshing feel.

- Raw Honey:
  - Raw honey is moisturizing and has antibacterial properties. It can help nourish the skin and promote a healthy glow.

- Tea Tree Essential Oil (Optional):
  - Tea tree oil is known for its antimicrobial properties, which can be beneficial for those with acne-prone skin.

**Note:** Perform a patch test before applying the mask to your face to ensure you don't have any adverse reactions to the ingredients. If you have sensitive skin, it's advisable to consult with a dermatologist before using a volcanic ash mask.

**Optional Additions:** Add yogurt, honey, or aloe vera gel based on your skin's needs. These additions can enhance the mask's soothing and moisturizing properties.

**Application:** Apply the mask evenly to cleansed skin, avoiding the eye area. Leave it on for 15-20 minutes or until the mask dries.

**Rinse:** Gently rinse off the mask with warm water, using circular motions to take advantage of the exfoliating properties.

**Moisturize:** Follow up with your favorite moisturizer to lock in hydration.

## Hibiscus Bath Soak

The Hibiscus Bath Soak offers a luxurious and aromatic experience, combining the beauty of dried hibiscus petals with the relaxation of a warm bath.

### Ingredients:

- Handful of dried hibiscus petals
- Epsom salt or sea salt

### Instructions:

1. Prepare the Bath: Fill your bathtub with warm water to your desired level.

2. Add Epsom Salt or Sea Salt: Pour a generous amount of Epsom salt or sea salt into the warm water. These salts help relax muscles and can contribute to a soothing bath experience.

3. Toss in Dried Hibiscus Petals: Take a handful of dried hibiscus petals and toss them into the bath. The vibrant color of the petals adds a visual appeal to the water, creating a beautiful and colorful soak.

4. Swirl and Mix: Gently swirl the water to help dissolve the salt and disperse the hibiscus petals throughout the bath.

5. Relax and Enjoy: Step into the bath, inhale the fragrant aroma of hibiscus, and immerse yourself in the soothing water. Close your eyes, take deep breaths, and let the combination of warm water and hibiscus petals relax your body and mind.

6. Optional Additions: For an extra touch of luxury, consider adding a few drops of your favorite essential oil or incorporating other botanicals like lavender buds or chamomile flowers.

7. Post-Bath Care: After your soak, pat your skin dry and moisturize to lock in hydration.

### Benefits:

- The hibiscus petals add a touch of elegance to your bath, creating a visually appealing and Instagram-worthy experience.
- Hibiscus is known for its soothing properties, making this bath soak ideal for relaxation and stress relief.
- Epsom salt or sea salt contributes to muscle relaxation and can help alleviate tension.

### History:

Bathing, especially with herbal-infused ingredients, has a rich history and is associated with various cultural and therapeutic benefits. Here's a brief overview of the historical benefits of bath soaks:

#### 1. Ancient Civilizations:
- Egypt: Ancient Egyptians were known for their love of bathing. They used a variety of oils, milk, and herbs in their baths for skincare and relaxation.
- Greece and Rome: Both ancient Greek and Roman cultures considered bathing a social activity. Public baths were places for socializing, exercise, and cleansing. Romans, in particular, used various oils, herbs, and flowers in their baths.

#### 2. Medieval Europe:
- In medieval Europe, public baths were popular, and herbs and flowers were added to bathwater for their perceived health benefits. Lavender, chamomile, and rosemary were common choices.

#### 3. Traditional Medicine:
- Traditional Chinese Medicine (TCM) and Ayurveda in India have long recommended herbal baths for their therapeutic effects. Various herbs were

chosen based on their properties, such as calming, detoxifying, or invigorating.

### 4. Renaissance Period:
- During the Renaissance, herbal baths became popular again. Lavender, rose, and chamomile were prized for their aromatic and relaxing qualities.

### 5. Victorian Era:
- In the Victorian era, the practice of bathing underwent a transformative shift, and herbs and perfumes played a pivotal role in shaping the bathing experience. As societal norms evolved and cleanliness became increasingly emphasized, individuals sought ways to make their bathing rituals not only hygienic but also luxurious and therapeutic.

Herbs like lavender, rose, and chamomile, celebrated for their aromatic qualities, were introduced into bathwater to infuse it with delightful scents. This incorporation of herbs served dual purposes—enhancing the bathing environment with pleasing fragrances and aligning with the Victorian belief in the healthful properties of botanicals.

These scented baths became synonymous with refinement and offered a sensory escape from the hustle of daily life. Moreover, the use of perfumes in bathing, whether in the form of scented oils or floral extracts, reflected a desire for elegance and an acknowledgment of the power of fragrance in uplifting the spirit. Victorian bathing, enriched by the infusion of herbs and perfumes, became a sensory indulgence and contributed to the ongoing tradition of associating self-care with delightful and aromatic experiences.

### 6. 20th Century and Beyond:
- With advancements in understanding aromatherapy and herbal medicine, the 20th century saw a resurgence of interest in herbal baths. People began recognizing the potential benefits of various herbs for relaxation, stress relief, and skin health.

### Historical Benefits:

- **Relaxation and Stress Relief:** Herbal baths were historically valued for their ability to promote relaxation and alleviate stress, both mentally and physically.
- **Skin Care:** Many herbs used in baths were chosen for their skincare properties. They were believed to cleanse, soothe, and nourish the skin.
- **Aromatherapy:** The aromatic qualities of herbs were often considered therapeutic. Different scents were believed to have different effects on mood and emotions.
- **Cultural and Social Practices:** Baths were not only about personal hygiene but also about socializing. Public baths in various cultures were gathering places for communities.

Today, the tradition of herbal-infused bathing continues, with people incorporating a variety of herbs, essential oils, and other natural ingredients into their bath rituals for both relaxation and skincare benefits.

**Note:** Ensure that you are not allergic to hibiscus before using it in your bath. If irritation occurs, discontinue use. Additionally, clean the bathtub thoroughly after use to prevent any staining from the hibiscus petals.

## Hibiscus-Lemon Foot Soak

This Hibiscus-Lemon Foot Soak is a simple yet effective way to pamper your feet, providing a refreshing and revitalizing foot spa experience. It's perfect for relieving tiredness after a long day or as part of a self-care routine. Adjust the quantities based on the size of your foot basin or bathtub.

### Ingredients:

- Warm water (enough to fill a foot basin or bathtub)
- Handful of dried hibiscus petals or one hibiscus tea bag
- 1 lemon
- Foot basin or bathtub

### Instructions:

1. Prepare Warm Water:
   - Fill a foot basin or bathtub with warm water. Ensure it's comfortable for soaking your feet.

2. Add Hibiscus Petals:
   - Drop a handful of dried hibiscus petals into the warm water. If using a tea bag, place it in the water.

3. Squeeze Lemon:
   - Squeeze the juice of one lemon into the water. You can also cut the lemon into slices and add them for an extra citrusy touch.

4. Mix Ingredients:
   - Gently stir the water to mix the hibiscus petals, lemon juice, and water.

5. Soak Your Feet:
   - Place your feet into the foot basin or bathtub and relax. Soak for 15-20 minutes, allowing the ingredients to work their magic.

6. Massage Your Feet:
   - While soaking, take the opportunity to massage your feet to enhance relaxation and stimulate blood circulation.

7. Pat Dry:
   - After soaking, pat your feet dry with a towel.

### Benefits:

A foot soak offers various benefits for both physical and mental well-being. Here are some of the advantages:

1. Relaxation and Stress Relief:
   - Soaking your feet in warm water is a calming experience that helps relax the muscles and alleviate stress. It can contribute to an overall sense of well-being and relaxation.

2. Improved Circulation:
   - Warm water helps dilate blood vessels, promoting better circulation. This can be especially beneficial for those who spend long hours on their feet or experience poor circulation.

3. Reduced Swelling and Inflammation:
   - A foot soak can help reduce swelling and inflammation in the feet and ankles, providing relief for individuals dealing with conditions like edema or after a long day of standing.

4. Pain Relief:
   - Warm water can soothe sore muscles and joints, offering relief from various foot ailments, including arthritis, plantar fasciitis, and general foot pain.

5. Hydration and Softening of Skin:
   - Soaking your feet in water helps hydrate the skin, preventing dryness and promoting softness. Adding moisturizing ingredients to the foot soak can enhance this effect.

6. Removal of Dead Skin Cells:
   - Soaking can help soften calluses and dead skin cells, making it easier to exfoliate and maintain healthy feet.

7. Improved Sleep:
   - The relaxation induced by a foot soak can contribute to better sleep quality. It's a simple and natural way to unwind before bedtime.

## Hibiscus Citrus Bliss Bath Crystals

This DIY Hibiscus Citrus Bliss Bath Crystals recipe offers a delightful and rejuvenating addition to your bath, combining the benefits of hibiscus, citrus, and essential oils for a blissful experience.

Ingredients:

- 1 cup Dead Sea salt
- 2 tablespoons hibiscus powder
- Zest of one citrus fruit (e.g., orange, grapefruit, or lemon)
- 10 drops grapefruit essential oil
- 10 drops orange essential oil
- 5 drops bergamot essential oil
- Mixing bowl
- Spoon
- Airtight container for storage

Instructions:

1. Prepare Citrus Zest:
   - Zest one citrus fruit (e.g., orange, grapefruit, or lemon). Ensure only the outer colored part is grated, avoiding the bitter white pith.

2. Combine Dry Ingredients:
   - In a mixing bowl, combine 1 cup of Dead Sea salt and 2 tablespoons of hibiscus powder. Mix well.

3. Add Citrus Zest:
   - Incorporate the citrus zest into the salt and hibiscus mixture. Stir thoroughly to distribute the zest evenly.

4. Introduce Essential Oils:
   - Add 10 drops of grapefruit essential oil, 10 drops of orange essential oil, and 5 drops of bergamot essential oil to the mixture. Mix well to ensure even distribution.

5. Mix Thoroughly:
   - Stir the ingredients thoroughly, ensuring that the essential oils are well combined with the salts and hibiscus.

6. Allow to Dry:
   - Spread the mixture on a flat surface or tray and allow it to dry completely. This process may take a few hours to a day, depending on the humidity in your environment.

7. Store in an Airtight Container:
   - Once dry, transfer the bath crystals into an airtight container for storage. This helps preserve the fragrance and quality of the crystals.

Abut Dead Sea Salt:
Derived from the Dead Sea, Dead Sea salt is a mineral-rich substance containing magnesium, calcium, potassium, and bromides. Known for its coarse texture, Dead Sea salt serves as an effective exfoliant, promoting skin renewal by removing dead cells.

With hygroscopic properties, it attracts and retains moisture, contributing to skin hydration and suppleness. The salt's minerals, particularly magnesium and bromides, are believed to soothe conditions like eczema and psoriasis. Additionally, Dead Sea salt is reputed for muscle relaxation and stress reduction during baths, cleansing properties that aid in detoxification, and its ability to balance skin pH.

When combined with essential oils, it enhances aromatherapy experiences, contributing to overall skin health with nourishing, cleansing, and rejuvenating properties.

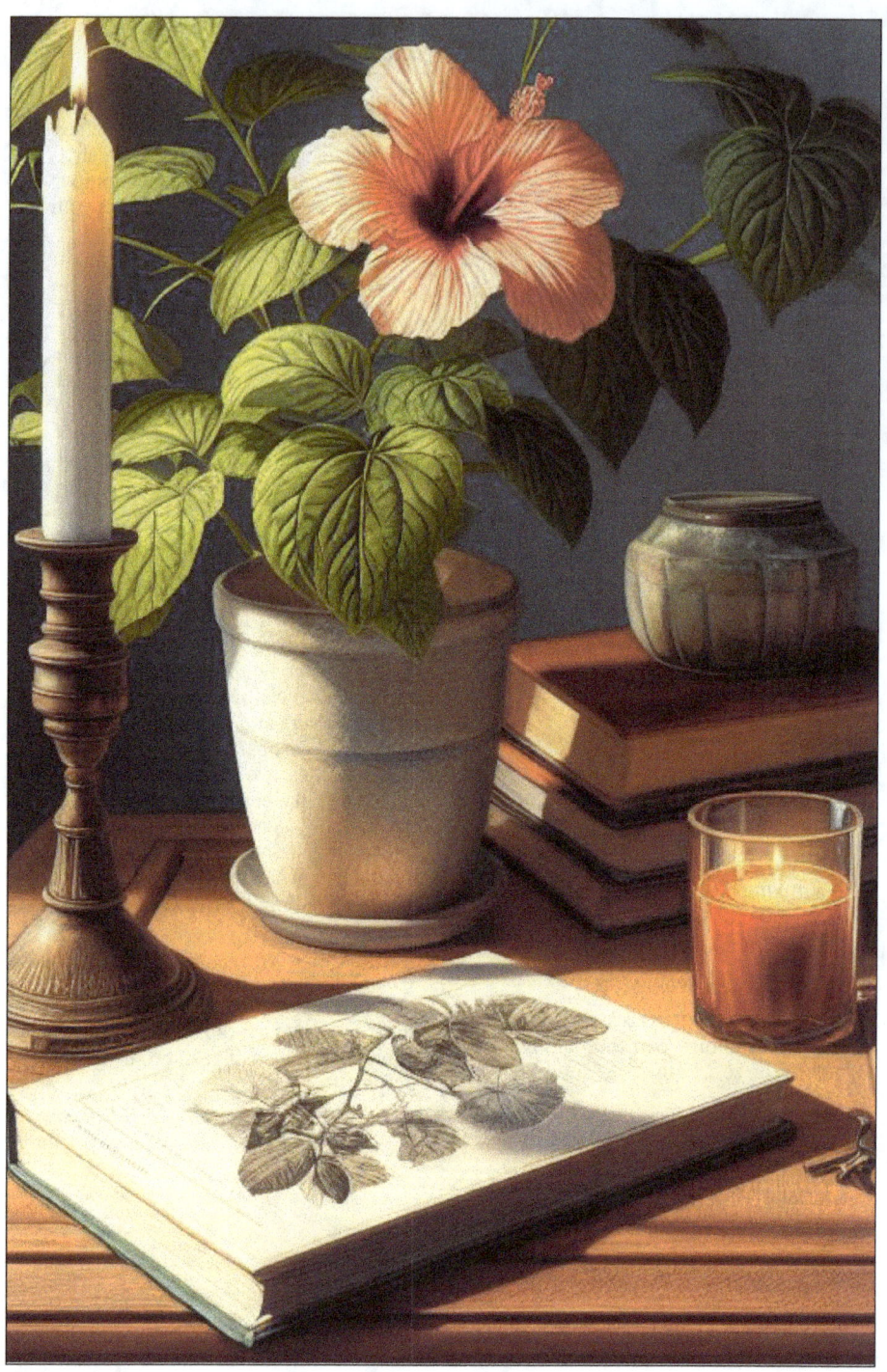

## Hibiscus Scented Candles

This DIY project results in a beautifully scented candle with the delightful addition of hibiscus petals.

### Materials:

- Soy wax flakes or blocks
- Hibiscus petals (dried)
- Fragrance oil (hibiscus-scented or your preferred floral scent)
- Wick with a metal base
- Wick holder or adhesive
- Double boiler or microwave-safe container
- Candle mold or container
- Stirring utensil
- Thermometer

### Instructions:

1. Prepare Your Work Area:
   - Cover your work surface with newspaper or a disposable tablecloth to catch any wax drips.

2. Measure Wax:
   - Determine the amount of wax needed based on the size of your candle container. Measure the wax flakes or blocks accordingly.

3. Melt the Wax:
   - Use a double boiler or a microwave-safe container to melt the soy wax. If using a microwave, heat in short intervals, stirring between each, until fully melted. Use a thermometer to monitor the temperature, and avoid overheating.

4. Add Fragrance Oil:
   - Once the wax is fully melted, add the hibiscus-scented fragrance oil. Follow the recommended usage guidelines on the fragrance oil packaging. Stir the wax thoroughly to distribute the fragrance.

5. Prepare the Wick:
   - Attach the metal base of the wick to the bottom center of your candle container using a wick holder or adhesive. Ensure the wick stands upright.

6. Secure the Wick:
   - Use a wick holder to keep the wick centered in the container as the wax solidifies. If you don't have a wick holder, you can fashion one using two pencils or chopsticks placed across the top of the container with the wick in between.

7. Add Hibiscus Petals:
   - Sprinkle a small amount of dried hibiscus petals into the bottom of the candle container. The petals will float within the candle as it solidifies.

8. Pour the Wax:
   - Carefully pour the melted wax into the container, leaving a small space at the top. Ensure the wick remains centered during this process.

9. Allow to Cool:
   - Let the candle cool and solidify completely. This may take several hours, depending on the size of the candle.

10. Trim the Wick:
    - Once the candle has hardened, trim the wick to your desired length, typically around half an inch above the wax surface.

11. Decorate (Optional):
    - If desired, you can further decorate the candle by placing additional hibiscus petals on the surface or tying a ribbon around the container.

12. Cure the Candle:
    - Allow the candle to cure for a day or two. This helps the fragrance develop and enhances the overall scent.

13. Light and Enjoy:
    - Your Hibiscus Scented Candle is ready to be lit! Enjoy the soothing aroma and the visual beauty of the hibiscus petals suspended within.

## Hibiscus and Jasmine Scented Milk Bath

This DIY Hibiscus and Jasmine Scented Milk Bath offers a decadent and moisturizing addition to your bath routine, combining the benefits of hibiscus, jasmine, oatmeal, and milk for a luxurious self-care experience.

Ingredients:

- 1/2 cup hibiscus powder
- 1/2 cup powdered jasmine flowers
- 1/4 cup colloidal oatmeal
- 1/2 cup whole milk powder
- Few drops of jasmine essential oil
- Mixing bowl
- Spoon
- Airtight container for storage

Instructions:

1. Combine Dry Ingredients:
   - In a mixing bowl, combine 1/2 cup of hibiscus powder, 1/2 cup of powdered jasmine flowers, 1/4 cup of colloidal oatmeal, and 1/2 cup of whole milk powder.

2. Mix Thoroughly:
   - Stir the dry ingredients together until well-blended, ensuring an even distribution of each component.

3. Add Jasmine Essential Oil:
   - Add a few drops of jasmine essential oil to the mixture. Adjust the amount based on your preference for scent intensity.

4. Mix Again:
   - Stir the mixture again to incorporate the jasmine essential oil, ensuring it is evenly distributed.

5. Transfer to Airtight Container:
   - Carefully transfer the scented milk bath mixture into an airtight container for storage. This helps preserve the fragrance and quality of the blend.

Usage:

1. Add to Bathwater:
   - Scoop 1/2 to 1 cup of the Hibiscus and Jasmine Scented Milk Bath mixture and add it to warm bathwater.

2. Dissolve in Water:
   - Allow the mixture to dissolve in the water, releasing the aromatic scents and nourishing properties.

3. Enjoy a Luxurious Bath:
   - Immerse yourself in the bath and enjoy a luxurious and moisturizing experience.

Benefits:

Jasmine Flowers:
   - Adds a delightful fragrance and potential skin-soothing properties.

Colloidal Oatmeal:
   - Colloidal oatmeal provides soothing and moisturizing benefits, helping to relieve dry or irritated skin. It forms a protective barrier, reducing inflammation and promoting skin comfort. With natural cleansing properties, colloidal oatmeal is often used to calm sensitive skin conditions and maintain a healthy skin barrier.

Whole Milk Powder:
   - Whole milk powder is a skincare ingredient that contains lactic acid, offering exfoliating and hydrating properties. It helps to nourish and soften the skin, promoting a smoother and more supple complexion. Additionally, the natural fats in whole milk powder contribute to skin moisture, making it a beneficial component in skincare formulations for those seeking hydration and improved skin texture.

Jasmine Essential Oil:
   - Enhances the sensory experience with a fragrant and calming aroma.

## Hibiscus Citrus Oatmeal Soap Bar

The Hibiscus Citrus Oatmeal Soap Bar is intended for use during regular bathing or showering. It offers a cleansing and refreshing experience, and the hibiscus petals and citrus aroma provide a touch of luxury to the skincare routine.

This soap can be a wonderful addition to your bathing routine, offering both visual appeal and a delightful sensory experience.

**Exfoliation:** The oatmeal base provides gentle exfoliation, promoting the removal of dead skin cells.

**Moisturization:** Sweet almond oil contributes to the soap's moisturizing properties, leaving the skin feeling soft.
Aromatherapy: The combination of hibiscus, citrus, and essential oils offers an aromatic experience that can be invigorating and uplifting.

### Ingredients:
- 1 cup oatmeal soap base
- 1 tablespoon dried hibiscus petals
- 1 tablespoon orange zest
- 1 teaspoon sweet almond oil
- 10-15 drops citrus essential oil (orange, lemon, or grapefruit)
- Soap mold

### Instructions:
1. Cut the oatmeal soap base into small cubes.
2. Melt the soap base in a double boiler or microwave-safe bowl.
3. Stir in the dried hibiscus petals, orange zest, sweet almond oil, and citrus essential oil.
4. Pour the mixture into the soap mold.
5. Allow the soap to cool and harden completely before removing from the mold.

## Hibiscus Bath Bomb

homemade bath bombs are relatively easy to make, and they offer a fun and customizable way to enhance your bath experience. Making bath bombs involves combining simple ingredients, molding them into shapes, and allowing them to dry.

### Ingredients:

- 1 cup baking soda
- 1/2 cup citric acid
- 1/2 cup cornstarch
- 1/4 cup Epsom salt
- 2 tablespoons dried hibiscus powder
- 1 tablespoon hibiscus-infused oil (coconut or sweet almond)
- 10-15 drops lavender essential oil (or your preferred scent)
- Witch hazel (in a spray bottle)

### Instructions:

1. In a bowl, mix together baking soda, citric acid, cornstarch, Epsom salt, and dried hibiscus powder.
2. In a separate bowl, combine the hibiscus-infused oil and essential oil.
3. Slowly add the liquid mixture to the dry ingredients, stirring constantly to avoid fizzing.
4. Spritz the mixture with witch hazel until it holds together when squeezed.
5. Pack the mixture into bath bomb molds or shape into balls.
6. Allow the bath bombs to dry and harden for at least 24 hours before use.

Enjoy these hibiscus-infused homemade soap bars and bath bomb for a luxurious and aromatic bathing experience!

# Hibiscus Household

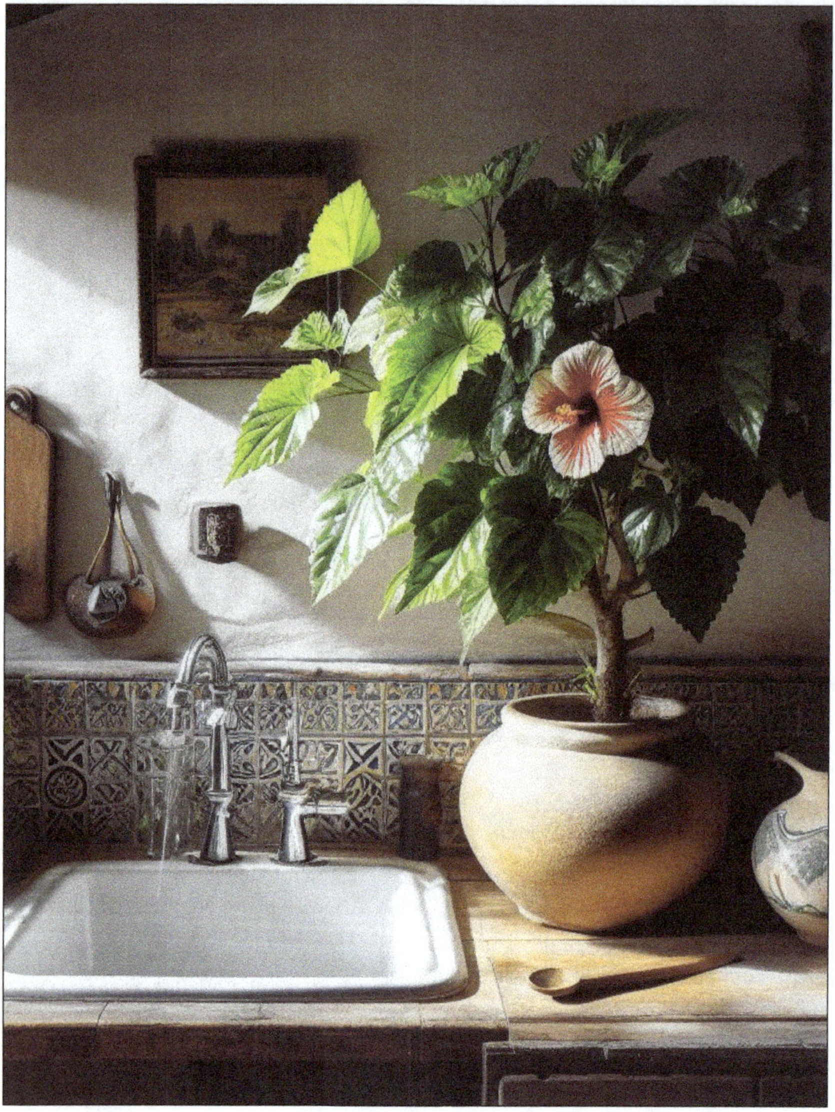

## Hibiscus All-Purpose Cleaner

This DIY hibiscus all-purpose cleaner provides an eco-friendly and aromatic alternative to commercial cleaners. The infused hibiscus adds a touch of natural fragrance while the vinegar and water combination effectively cleans and disinfects various surfaces in your home.

The Hibiscus All-Purpose Cleaner is a natural and fragrant cleaning solution that harnesses the cleaning properties of white vinegar along with the pleasant aroma and potential antibacterial benefits of hibiscus petals. Here's a brief overview of how to make and use this cleaner:

### Ingredients:

1. White Vinegar: Known for its disinfectant properties and ability to break down grease and grime.

2. Water: Helps dilute the solution and create a balance for effective cleaning.

3. Hibiscus Petals: Apart from adding a pleasant fragrance, hibiscus petals may contribute some antibacterial and antiviral properties.

### Instructions:

1. Infusing the Hibiscus:
   - In a clean glass jar, combine a handful of dried hibiscus petals with white vinegar. Seal the jar and let it sit for at least a week, allowing the hibiscus to infuse into the vinegar.

2. Creating the Cleaner:
   - Strain the infused vinegar to remove the hibiscus petals, leaving behind a hibiscus-infused vinegar. Mix this infused vinegar with an equal amount of water. The result is your hibiscus all-purpose cleaner.

3. Application:
   - Transfer the cleaner to a spray bottle for easy application. Shake well before use to ensure even distribution.

4. Cleaning Surfaces:
   - Use the hibiscus all-purpose cleaner on various surfaces such as countertops, kitchen appliances, bathroom fixtures, and more. Spray directly onto the surface and wipe with a clean cloth or sponge.

5. Fragrance Boost:
   - Enjoy the natural and floral fragrance of the hibiscus cleaner as it leaves surfaces clean and refreshed.

### Additional Tips:

- **Storage:** Store the hibiscus all-purpose cleaner in a cool, dark place when not in use.

- **Experiment with Ratios:** Adjust the ratio of hibiscus-infused vinegar to water based on your preference for a more concentrated or milder cleaner.

- **Customization:** Consider adding a few drops of essential oils, such as lavender or tea tree oil, for added cleaning power and a personalized scent.

## Hibiscus Linen Spray

Hibiscus linen spray provides a natural and aromatic touch to your living spaces, adding a hint of floral freshness to your linens and surroundings. It's a simple yet effective DIY project that brings the soothing qualities of hibiscus into your daily life.

Hibiscus Linen Spray is a simple and delightful way to add a burst of natural fragrance to your linens, bedding, and even the air in your living spaces. Here's a brief guide on how to make and use it:

### Ingredients:

1. Hibiscus-Infused Water: Prepare by steeping dried hibiscus petals in water until the water is infused with the floral essence.

2. Essential Oil (Optional): Choose a complementary essential oil for added fragrance. Lavender, chamomile, or ylang-ylang work well.

### Instructions:

1. Prepare Hibiscus-Infused Water:
   - Steep a handful of dried hibiscus petals in water. Allow the petals to infuse for several hours or overnight. Strain the petals, leaving behind the hibiscus-infused water.

2. Add Essential Oil (Optional):
   - If you desire a more complex fragrance, add a few drops of your chosen essential oil to the hibiscus-infused water. Essential oils like lavender or chamomile can complement the hibiscus scent.

3. Pour into a Spray Bottle:
   - Transfer the hibiscus-infused water (with or without essential oil) into a clean and empty spray bottle. A funnel can be helpful for this step.

4. Shake Well:
   - Shake the spray bottle well to ensure the hibiscus-infused water and essential oil are thoroughly mixed.

5. Application:
   - Lightly mist the hibiscus linen spray onto your linens, pillows, curtains, or even into the air for a refreshing burst of natural fragrance.

6. Allow to Dry:
   - After spraying, allow the linens to air dry. The hibiscus linen spray will leave behind a subtle and pleasant aroma.

### Tips:

- **Storage:** Store the hibiscus linen spray in a cool, dark place when not in use. Shake well before each use to disperse the fragrance evenly.

- **Experiment with Scents:** Feel free to experiment with different essential oils to create a customized fragrance blend that suits your preferences.

- **Relaxation Ritual:** Use the hibiscus linen spray as part of your bedtime routine to create a calming and soothing atmosphere in your bedroom.

# Hibiscus Dish Soap

Creating hibiscus dish soap adds a touch of natural beauty and fragrance to a typically mundane task. The infusion of hibiscus offers not only a pleasant aroma but potentially some additional benefits for your skin. Enjoy the beauty of this floral dish soap as you make your daily chores more enjoyable.

Here's a simple guide on how to make it:

### Ingredients:

1. Liquid Castile Soap: A plant-based soap that serves as the base for your dish soap.

2. Dried Hibiscus Petals: For both visual appeal and potential additional properties.

3. Essential Oil (Optional): Choose a mild and complementary essential oil such as lavender or lemon for fragrance.

### Instructions:

1. Prepare Hibiscus-Infused Soap Base:
   - Heat the liquid castile soap on low heat until it's warm. Add a handful of dried hibiscus petals to the warm soap and let it steep for a few hours or overnight.

2. Strain the Petals:
   - Strain the hibiscus-infused soap to remove the petals, leaving behind a soap base infused with the floral essence.

3. Add Essential Oil (Optional):
   - If you desire additional fragrance, add a few drops of essential oil to the hibiscus-infused soap. Stir well to ensure even distribution.

4. Transfer to a Dispenser:
   - Pour the hibiscus-infused soap into a clean and empty dish soap dispenser. A funnel can be useful for this step.

5. Usage:
   - Use the hibiscus dish soap as you would any regular dish soap. Dispense a small amount onto a sponge or directly onto dishes, and wash as usual.

6. Enjoy the Floral Touch:
   - Experience the subtle floral fragrance and the visual appeal of the hibiscus-infused dish soap as you wash your dishes.

### Tips:

- **Storage:** Store the hibiscus dish soap in a cool place when not in use. Shake well before each use to ensure the hibiscus essence is evenly distributed.

- **Experiment with Strength:** Adjust the concentration of hibiscus-infused soap based on your preferences for a milder or stronger floral scent.

- **Mild Essential Oils:** If adding essential oils, choose oils that are gentle and suitable for dishwashing.

## Hibiscus Carpet Freshener

This DIY hibiscus carpet freshener not only neutralizes odors but also brings a touch of nature into your home. The combination of baking soda, hibiscus, and optional essential oils provides an effective and aromatic solution for keeping your carpets and rugs smelling clean and inviting.

### Ingredients:

1. Baking Soda: Known for its odor-absorbing properties.

2. Dried Hibiscus Petals: Adds a visually appealing touch and imparts a pleasant fragrance.

3. Essential Oil (Optional): Choose a complementary essential oil, such as lavender or eucalyptus, for added fragrance.

### Instructions:

1. Prepare Hibiscus-Infused Baking Soda:
   - In a bowl, mix baking soda with a handful of dried hibiscus petals. Allow the mixture to sit for a few hours or overnight to let the hibiscus infuse into the baking soda.

2. Strain the Petals:
   - After the hibiscus has infused into the baking soda, strain the mixture to remove the petals, leaving behind hibiscus-infused baking soda.

3. Add Essential Oil (Optional):
   - If you want to enhance the fragrance, add a few drops of your chosen essential oil to the hibiscus-infused baking soda. Mix well.

4. Transfer to a Shaker Container:
   - Pour the hibiscus-infused baking soda into a shaker container. This can be a recycled spice container or any container with a shaker top.

5. Application:
   - Sprinkle the hibiscus carpet freshener liberally over your carpet or rug.

6. Wait and Vacuum:
   - Let the hibiscus-infused baking soda sit on the carpet for at least 15-20 minutes to allow it to absorb odors. Afterward, vacuum thoroughly to remove the baking soda.

7. Enjoy Freshened Carpets:
   - Experience the subtle floral fragrance that lingers on your carpets, creating a refreshed and pleasant atmosphere.

### Tips:

- **Storage:** Store any leftover hibiscus carpet freshener in a cool, dry place.

- **Experiment with Scents:** Feel free to experiment with different essential oils to create a customized fragrance blend that suits your preferences.

- **Regular Use:** Use the hibiscus carpet freshener as needed to keep your carpets smelling fresh.

## Hibiscus Furniture Polish

This DIY hibiscus furniture polish offers a natural and aromatic alternative to commercial furniture polishes. The combination of hibiscus-infused oil, white vinegar, and optional essential oils not only cleans and shines but also adds a touch of nature to your home.

Ingredients:

1. Olive Oil or Jojoba Oil: Provides a natural and nourishing base for the polish.

2. White Vinegar: Helps clean and remove any residues from the furniture.

3. Dried Hibiscus Petals: Adds a visually appealing touch and may contribute a subtle fragrance.

4. Essential Oil (Optional): Choose a wood-friendly essential oil like lemon or cedar for added fragrance.

Instructions:

1. Prepare Hibiscus-Infused Oil:
 - Heat olive oil or jojoba oil on low heat. Add a handful of dried hibiscus petals to the warm oil and let it steep for several hours or overnight.

2. Strain the Petals:
 - Strain the hibiscus-infused oil to remove the petals, leaving behind hibiscus-infused oil.

3. Mix with White Vinegar:
 - In a bowl, combine the hibiscus-infused oil with an equal amount of white vinegar. The vinegar helps clean and degrease the furniture.

4. Add Essential Oil (Optional):
 - If you wish to enhance the fragrance, add a few drops of your chosen wood-friendly essential oil. Stir well.

5. Transfer to a Container:
 - Pour the hibiscus furniture polish into a clean and empty container, preferably one with a lid.

6. Application:
 - Dip a soft, lint-free cloth into the hibiscus furniture polish. Apply it evenly to your wooden furniture, working with the grain.

7. Buff to Shine:
 - After applying the polish, buff the furniture with a clean, dry cloth to bring out a natural shine.

8. Enjoy Lustrous Furniture:
 - Experience the revitalized and subtly fragrant appearance of your wooden furniture.

Tips:

- **Storage:** Store the hibiscus furniture polish in a cool, dark place when not in use.

- **Regular Use:** Use the polish regularly to maintain the shine and condition of your wooden furniture.

- **Wood-Friendly Essential Oils:** When choosing essential oils, opt for scents that complement wood and are suitable for furniture, such as citrus or woodsy oils.

## Hibiscus Stain Remover

This DIY hibiscus stain remover provides a natural and gentle solution for tackling stains on fabrics. The combination of hibiscus-infused water, liquid dish soap, and optional baking soda offers an effective and eco-friendly way to lift and remove various types of stains.

### Ingredients:

1. Hibiscus-Infused Water: Prepared by steeping dried hibiscus petals in water.

2. Liquid Dish Soap: Mild dish soap helps break down and lift stains.

3. Baking Soda (Optional): Acts as a gentle abrasive to aid in stain removal.

### Instructions:

1. Prepare Hibiscus-Infused Water:
   - Steep a handful of dried hibiscus petals in warm water until the water is infused with the floral essence. Allow the mixture to cool.

2. Mix with Dish Soap:
   - In a bowl, combine the hibiscus-infused water with a small amount of liquid dish soap. Stir well to create a soapy solution.

3. Add Baking Soda (Optional):
   - If dealing with a tougher stain, you can add a pinch of baking soda to the mixture. Baking soda acts as a gentle abrasive to help lift stains.

4. Apply to Stain:
   - Dab a clean cloth or sponge into the hibiscus stain remover mixture. Gently blot or rub the stained area with the solution.

5. Let it Sit:
   - Allow the hibiscus stain remover to sit on the stain for a few minutes. This gives the solution time to break down and lift the stain.

6. Blot or Rinse:
   - Blot the stained area with a clean, damp cloth or rinse the fabric under cold water to remove the stain and any residue.

7. Check the Stain:
   - Check the stain. If needed, repeat the process until the stain is fully removed.

8. Wash as Usual:
   - After treating the stain, wash the fabric as usual to remove any remaining traces of the stain remover.

### Tips:

- **Test on a Small Area:** Before applying the hibiscus stain remover to a visible area, test it on a small, inconspicuous part of the fabric to ensure compatibility.

- **Adjust Ingredients:** Depending on the type of stain, you can adjust the amount of dish soap or add baking soda for more abrasive action.

- **Immediate Treatment:** For best results, treat stains as soon as possible after they occur.

# Hibiscus Pot and Pan Scrub

This DIY hibiscus pot and pan scrub offers a natural and effective solution for cleaning cookware. The combination of ground hibiscus petals, baking soda, and dish soap provides a gentle abrasive action, making it suitable for various types of pots and pans.

### Ingredients:

1. Dried Hibiscus Petals: Adds a natural and visually appealing element.

2. Baking Soda: Acts as a gentle abrasive to help scrub away residues.

3. Liquid Dish Soap: Provides additional cleaning power.

### Instructions:

1. Grind Dried Hibiscus Petals:
   - Use a mortar and pestle or a grinder to grind the dried hibiscus petals into a coarse powder.

2. Mix with Baking Soda:
   - In a bowl, combine the ground hibiscus petals with baking soda. Adjust the ratio based on the level of abrasiveness you desire.

3. Add Liquid Dish Soap:
   - Add a small amount of liquid dish soap to the dry mixture. Stir well to create a paste. The dish soap enhances the scrubbing power.

4. Apply to Cookware:
   - Dampen the surface of your pot or pan, then apply the hibiscus scrub paste. Use a sponge, scrub brush, or cloth to scrub the surface.

5. Scrub Thoroughly:
   - Focus on areas with stains or residues, scrubbing thoroughly to lift and remove them.

6. Rinse with Water:
   - Rinse the cookware with water to remove the scrub residue.

7. Enjoy Clean Cookware:
   - Experience the results of clean and refreshed pots and pans.

### Tips:

- **Test on a Small Area:** Before applying the hibiscus scrub to the entire cookware, test it on a small, inconspicuous area to ensure compatibility.

- **Adjust Ingredients:** Depending on the type of cookware and the intensity of cleaning needed, you can adjust the ratio of hibiscus petals, baking soda, and dish soap.

- **Regular Maintenance:** Use the hibiscus pot and pan scrub regularly to maintain the cleanliness of your cookware.

## Hibiscus Deodorizing Bags

These DIY hibiscus deodorizing bags provide a natural and visually appealing solution to keep small spaces smelling fresh. The combination of hibiscus petals and baking soda helps eliminate odors while imparting a pleasant fragrance.

### Ingredients:

1. Dried Hibiscus Petals: Adds a visually appealing and fragrant element.

2. Baking Soda: Acts as a natural deodorizer to absorb and neutralize odors.

3. Small Fabric Bags or Sachets: Provides a container for the deodorizing mixture.

### Instructions:

1. Prepare the Deodorizing Mixture:
   - In a bowl, mix dried hibiscus petals with baking soda. The hibiscus adds fragrance, while baking soda helps eliminate odors.

2. Fill Fabric Bags:
   - Fill small fabric bags or sachets with the hibiscus and baking soda mixture. Tie or seal the bags securely.

3. Place in Small Spaces:
   - Put the hibiscus deodorizing bags in small spaces where odors may linger, such as closets, drawers, shoes, or gym bags.

4. Replace as Needed:
   - Over time, the baking soda may lose its effectiveness. Replace or refresh the hibiscus deodorizing bags every few weeks or as needed.

5. Enjoy Natural Freshness:
   - Experience the subtle hibiscus fragrance and the natural deodorizing properties of the baking soda in your small spaces.

### Tips:

- **Essential Oils (Optional):** If you desire a stronger fragrance, you can add a few drops of essential oil, such as lavender or tea tree oil, to the hibiscus and baking soda mixture.

- **Sun Exposure:** Occasionally place the deodorizing bags in direct sunlight to help refresh the hibiscus and baking soda.

- **Storage:** When not in use, store the hibiscus deodorizing bags in a cool, dry place to maintain their effectiveness.

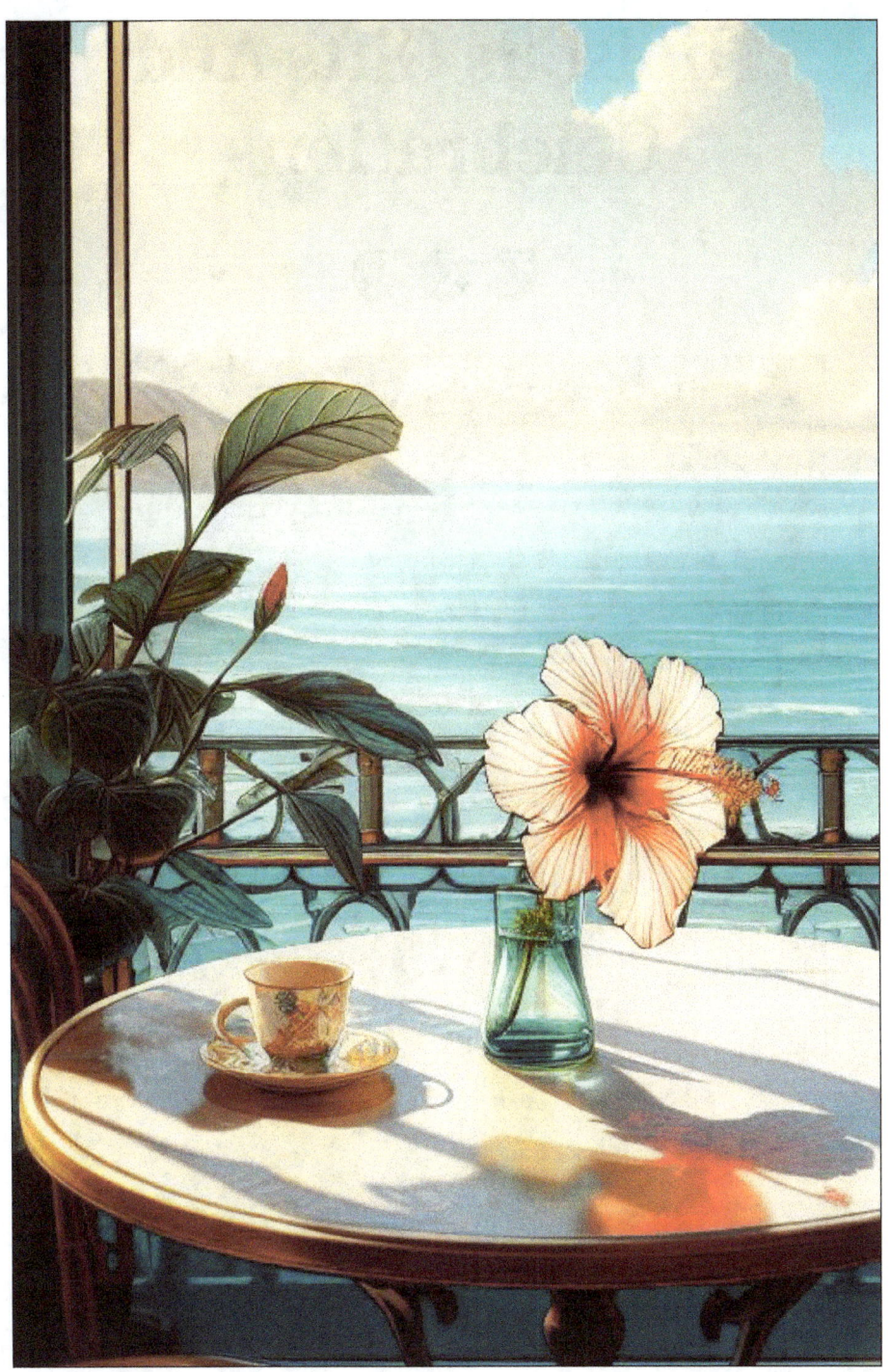

# Hibiscus Gifts And Celebrations

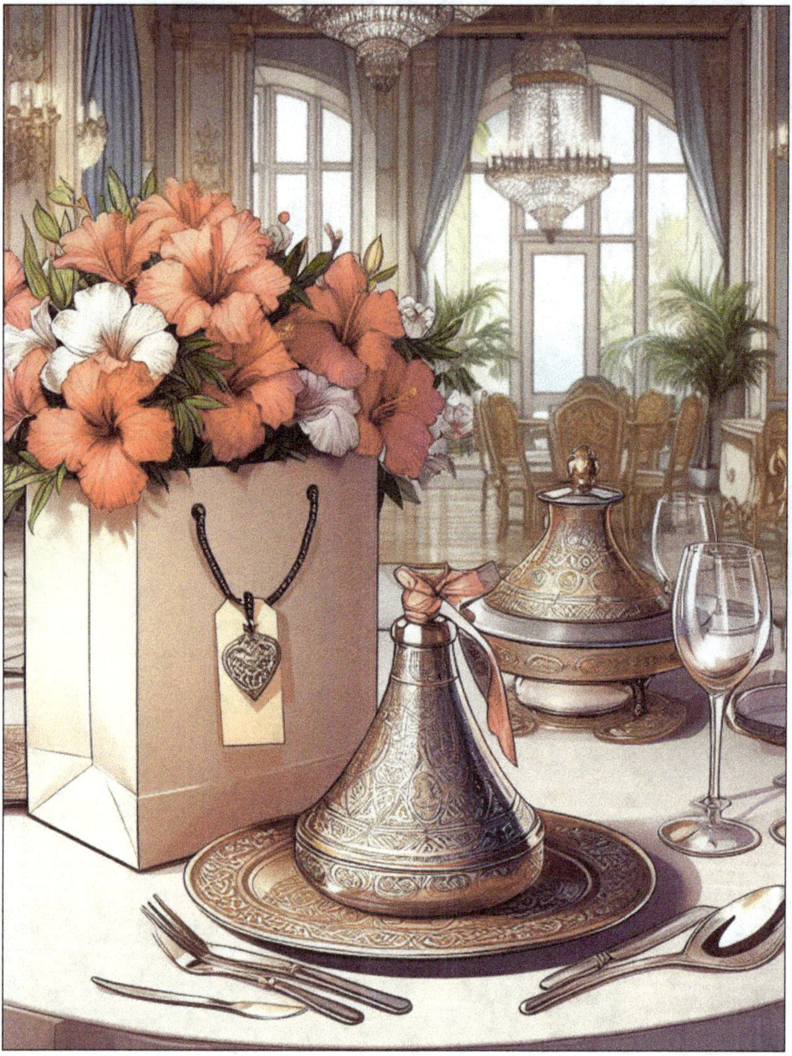

## Hibiscus-Scented Cologne

Creating your own hibiscus-scented cologne not only provides a personalized fragrance but also allows you to enjoy the natural and floral essence of hibiscus.

### Ingredients:

1. Dried Hibiscus Petals: 2-3 tablespoons
2. High-Quality Vodka or Witch Hazel: 1 cup
3. Distilled Water: 1/2 cup
4. Essential Oils: Optional for additional fragrance (suggestions: bergamot, cedarwood, or lavender)
5. Dark Glass Bottle: To store the cologne
6. Funnel and Cheesecloth or Fine Mesh Strainer: For straining the mixture

### Instructions:

1. Prepare the Hibiscus Infusion:
   - In a clean glass jar, combine the dried hibiscus petals with vodka or witch hazel. Seal the jar and let it sit in a cool, dark place for about two weeks to allow the hibiscus to infuse into the alcohol.

2. Strain the Mixture:
   - After two weeks, strain the hibiscus-infused liquid using a funnel and cheesecloth or a fine mesh strainer to remove the petals. Discard the used petals.

3. Add Distilled Water:
   - Mix the hibiscus-infused alcohol with distilled water. This helps balance the strength of the cologne and adds a refreshing touch.

4. Optional: Add Essential Oils:
   - If you desire a more complex fragrance, add a few drops of essential oils. Start with a small amount and adjust to your preference. Essential oils like bergamot, cedarwood, or lavender can complement the hibiscus scent.

5. Test and Adjust:
   - Test the cologne on your wrist and adjust the fragrance or strength by adding more distilled water or essential oils as needed.

6. Store in a Dark Glass Bottle:
   - Pour the hibiscus-scented cologne into a dark glass bottle using a funnel. Dark glass helps protect the cologne from light, preserving its fragrance.

7. Let it Mature:
   - Allow the cologne to mature for at least a week in the bottle. This gives the ingredients time to blend and develop a well-rounded scent.

8. Application:
   - Apply the hibiscus-scented cologne to pulse points, such as wrists and neck, for a subtle and long-lasting fragrance.

### Tips:

- **Experiment with Ratios:** Adjust the ratio of hibiscus infusion, water, and essential oils to achieve the desired strength and fragrance.

- **Personalize the Scent:** Play around with different essential oil combinations to create a unique and personalized fragrance.

- **Store Properly:** Keep the cologne in a cool, dark place to preserve its scent. Shake the bottle before each use to mix the ingredients.

## Hibiscus Shaving Cream

Creating your own hibiscus-infused shaving cream provides a natural and delightful addition to your grooming routine. The combination of hibiscus, coconut oil, and shea butter offers a nourishing and aromatic experience for a smooth shave.

### Ingredients:

1. Dried Hibiscus Petals: 2-3 tablespoons
2. Coconut Oil: 1/2 cup
3. Shea Butter: 1/4 cup
4. Jojoba Oil: 2 tablespoons
5. Liquid Castile Soap: 1 tablespoon
6. Essential Oils: Optional for fragrance (suggestions: peppermint, eucalyptus, or lavender)
7. Distilled Water: 1/4 cup
8. Double Boiler or Microwave-Safe Bowl
9. Hand Mixer or Blender
10. Sealable Container or Jar: To store the shaving cream

### Instructions:

1. Prepare the Hibiscus Infusion:
   - In a double boiler or microwave-safe bowl, melt coconut oil. Add dried hibiscus petals and let them infuse into the melted coconut oil. Allow it to cool and strain to remove the petals.

2. Melt Shea Butter:
   - Melt the shea butter in the double boiler or microwave-safe bowl along with the hibiscus-infused coconut oil.

3. Add Jojoba Oil and Castile Soap:
   - Mix in jojoba oil and liquid castile soap to the melted oils. Stir well to combine.

4. Optional: Add Essential Oils:
   - If desired, add a few drops of essential oils for fragrance. Peppermint, eucalyptus, or lavender are popular choices.

5. Cooling Phase:
   - Allow the mixture to cool for a while but not to the point of solidifying.

6. Blending:
   - Use a hand mixer or blender to whip the cooled mixture until it reaches a creamy and smooth consistency.

7. Add Distilled Water:
   - Gradually add distilled water while continuing to whip the mixture. This step helps achieve a lighter and fluffier texture.

8. Store in Container:
   - Transfer the hibiscus shaving cream to a sealable container or jar. Store in a cool place.

9. Application:
   - Apply the shaving cream to damp skin before shaving. Enjoy the nourishing and aromatic experience.

### Tips:

- **Test Sensitivity:** Before regular use, test a small amount of the shaving cream on a patch of skin to ensure there's no sensitivity or irritation.

- **Customize Fragrance:** Experiment with different essential oil combinations to create a personalized fragrance profile.

- **Shelf Life:** Store the shaving cream in a cool place. If you notice any changes in texture or scent, consider making smaller batches for freshness.

## Hibiscus Perfume

This DIY hibiscus-scented perfume is a lovely and personalized gift that captures the essence of hibiscus in a beautiful fragrance.

### Ingredients:

1. Dried Hibiscus Petals: 2-3 tablespoons
2. High-Quality Vodka or Jojoba Oil: 1 cup
3. Distilled Water: 1/2 cup
4. Essential Oils: Optional for additional fragrance (suggestions: jasmine, rose, or vanilla)
5. Dark Glass Perfume Bottle: To store the perfume
6. Funnel and Cheesecloth or Fine Mesh Strainer: For straining the mixture

### Instructions:

1. Prepare the Hibiscus Infusion:
   - In a clean glass jar, combine the dried hibiscus petals with vodka or jojoba oil. Seal the jar and let it sit in a cool, dark place for about two weeks to allow the hibiscus to infuse into the alcohol or oil.

2. Strain the Mixture:
   - After two weeks, strain the hibiscus-infused liquid using a funnel and cheesecloth or a fine mesh strainer to remove the petals. Discard the used petals.

3. Add Distilled Water:
   - Mix the hibiscus-infused alcohol or oil with distilled water. This helps balance the strength of the perfume and adds a refreshing touch. For oil-based perfumes, you can skip this step if you prefer a more concentrated scent.

4. Optional: Add Essential Oils:
   - If you desire a more complex fragrance, add a few drops of essential oils. Start with a small amount and adjust to your preference. Essential oils like jasmine, rose, or vanilla can complement the hibiscus scent beautifully.

5. Test and Adjust:
   - Test the perfume on your wrist and adjust the fragrance or strength by adding more distilled water or essential oils as needed.

6. Store in a Dark Glass Bottle:
   - Pour the hibiscus-scented perfume into a dark glass bottle using a funnel. Dark glass helps protect the perfume from light, preserving its fragrance.

7. Let it Mature:
   - Allow the perfume to mature for at least a week in the bottle. This gives the ingredients time to blend and develop a well-rounded scent.

8. Application:
   - Apply the hibiscus-scented perfume to pulse points, such as wrists and neck, for a beautifully scented experience.

### Tips:

- **Experiment with Ratios:** Adjust the ratio of hibiscus infusion, water, and essential oils to achieve the desired strength and fragrance.

- **Personalize the Scent:** Play around with different essential oil combinations to create a unique and personalized fragrance that she'll love.

- **Gift Presentation:** Consider presenting the perfume in a decorated bottle or box for a special touch.

# Hibiscus-Infused Chocolate Truffles

Chocolate truffles are decadent and luxurious confections that consist of a creamy ganache center coated in various outer layers.

These truffles are a sublime fusion of rich dark chocolate and the delicate, floral notes of hibiscus. The process begins with the infusion of heavy cream with dried hibiscus petals, imparting a subtle and enchanting floral essence. The hibiscus-infused cream is then blended with finely chopped dark chocolate until a velvety ganache is achieved. This luscious ganache is allowed to cool and set, transforming into a smooth and indulgent filling.

Each truffle is meticulously handcrafted into bite-sized orbs of pure delight. Their outer layer, a dusting of cocoa powder, provides a touch of bitterness that beautifully complements the sweet and floral interior. The truffles are then elegantly presented, nestled in mini cupcake liners, creating a visually appealing and romantic display.

With each bite, the hibiscus-infused chocolate truffle offers a symphony of flavors – the rich, melt-in-your-mouth chocolate, the subtle floral undertones of hibiscus, and the satisfying cocoa dusting that lingers on the palate. These truffles are not merely sweets; they are an exquisite expression of love and sophistication, making them a perfect gift or a treat for special occasions.

## Hibiscus and Orange Zest Chocolate Truffles

Ingredients:
- Dark chocolate (70% cocoa)
- Heavy cream
- Dried hibiscus petals
- Orange zest
- Cocoa powder for dusting

Instructions:
1. Heat the heavy cream until it simmers.
2. Steep dried hibiscus petals and orange zest in the hot cream for 15 minutes.
3. Strain the cream to remove the petals and zest and reheat.
4. Pour the hot cream over finely chopped dark chocolate, stirring until smooth.
5. Chill the mixture until it's firm enough to scoop.
6. Form the mixture into small truffle-sized balls and roll them in cocoa powder.
7. Place the truffles in mini cupcake liners for a delightful presentation.

## Hibiscus and Edible Gold Leaf Chocolate Truffles

Ingredients:
- Dark chocolate (70% cocoa)
- Heavy cream
- Dried hibiscus petals
- Edible gold leaf sheets
- Cocoa powder for dusting

Instructions:
1. Heat the heavy cream until it simmers.
2. Steep dried hibiscus petals in the hot cream for 15 minutes.
3. Strain the cream to remove the petals and reheat.
4. Pour the hot cream over finely chopped dark chocolate, stirring until smooth.
5. Chill the mixture until it's firm enough to scoop.
6. Carefully wrap a small piece of edible gold leaf around each truffle.
7. Form the mixture into small truffle-sized balls and dust them lightly with cocoa powder.
8. Place the truffles in mini cupcake liners for a luxurious presentation.

The second version incorporates edible gold leaf, which is an elegant and expensive touch, perfect for special occasions like Valentine's Day. These truffles not only taste exquisite but also offer a visually stunning and luxurious treat for your loved one.

## Grilled Hibiscus-Glazed Chicken Skewers with Pineapple Mango Salsa

This informal and fun Pacific Island-inspired dish brings together the floral notes of hibiscus with the tropical sweetness of pineapple and mango. The grilled chicken skewers, glazed with a hibiscus-infused sauce, paired with the vibrant fruit salsa, create a delightful and exotic culinary experience.

### Ingredients:

For the Hibiscus-Glazed Chicken Skewers:
- 1.5 lbs boneless, skinless chicken thighs, cut into cubes
- 1/2 cup hibiscus tea (brewed and cooled)
- 1/4 cup soy sauce
- 1/4 cup honey
- 2 tablespoons sesame oil
- 2 cloves garlic, minced
- 1 teaspoon grated ginger
- Wooden skewers, soaked in water

For the Pineapple Mango Salsa:
- 1 cup diced pineapple
- 1 cup diced mango
- 1/4 cup red onion, finely chopped
- 1 jalapeño, seeded and minced
- 2 tablespoons fresh cilantro, chopped
- Juice of 1 lime
- Salt and pepper to taste

### Instructions:

1. Hibiscus-Glazed Chicken Skewers:
1. In a bowl, whisk together hibiscus tea, soy sauce, honey, sesame oil, minced garlic, and grated ginger to create the glaze.
2. Thread the chicken cubes onto the soaked wooden skewers.
3. Place the skewers in a shallow dish and pour half of the glaze over them. Marinate for at least 30 minutes.
4. Preheat the grill to medium-high heat.
5. Grill the chicken skewers for about 5-7 minutes per side, basting with the remaining glaze, until the chicken is fully cooked and has a glossy glaze.

2. Pineapple Mango Salsa:
1. In a bowl, combine diced pineapple, diced mango, finely chopped red onion, minced jalapeño, chopped cilantro, lime juice, salt, and pepper.
2. Gently toss the ingredients together and refrigerate for at least 15 minutes.

3. Assembling:
1. Arrange the Grilled Hibiscus-Glazed Chicken Skewers on a serving platter.
2. Spoon Pineapple Mango Salsa over the top of each skewer.
3. Garnish with additional cilantro and lime wedges.

## Moroccan-Inspired Hibiscus-Infused Chicken Tagine

Embark on a culinary voyage with our exquisite Hibiscus-Infused Chicken Tagine, a dish inspired by the rich and diverse flavors of Moroccan cuisine. In this gastronomic masterpiece, succulent bone-in, skin-on chicken thighs are marinated in a symphony of spices and the floral elegance of hibiscus tea. Slow-cooked to perfection in a traditional tagine, the result is a tender and aromatic masterpiece that captures the essence of Moroccan culinary artistry.

### Historical Nuances:
Moroccan cuisine, with its centuries-old traditions, has been shaped by the confluence of diverse cultures. The spices, such as cumin, coriander, cinnamon, and turmeric, reflect the historical influences of Arab, Berber, and Mediterranean culinary heritage. The use of the tagine, a traditional earthenware pot, adds authenticity to this dish, as it has been an integral part of Moroccan cooking for centuries.

### Hibiscus Inclusion:
The infusion of hibiscus in this tagine is a nod to Morocco's historical trade connections with regions where hibiscus is cultivated. Known for its vibrant color and subtle floral notes, hibiscus elevates the dish, providing a unique twist to traditional flavors. Beyond its aesthetic appeal, hibiscus also brings a hint of tartness, balancing the richness of the chicken and adding depth to the culinary experience.

### Perfect for a Formal Celebration:
This Hibiscus-Infused Chicken Tagine is more than a dish; it's a celebration on a plate, making it the perfect centerpiece for formal occasions among friends or loved ones. The slow-cooked chicken, tender and infused with the exotic blend of spices and hibiscus, is a testament to the care and craftsmanship put into Moroccan culinary traditions.

### Reasons to Choose this Dish:

1. **Elegance:** The tagine's presentation, with its conical lid and vibrant colors, adds a touch of elegance to any formal gathering.
2. **Complex Flavors:** The intricate blend of spices and the floral infusion of hibiscus create a symphony of flavors that will delight the palate.
3. **Shared Experience:** Moroccan cuisine is inherently communal, making this dish ideal for sharing and fostering a sense of togetherness.

In summary, our Hibiscus-Infused Chicken Tagine is a celebration of history, flavor, and shared experiences. It embodies the essence of Moroccan culinary heritage, making it the perfect choice for a formal celebratory event where friends and loved ones can come together to savor the richness of tradition and the joy of shared moments.

### Ingredients:

**For the Hibiscus-Infused Chicken Tagine:**
- 2 lbs bone-in, skin-on chicken thighs
- 1 cup hibiscus tea (brewed and cooled)
- 1 large onion, finely chopped
- 3 cloves garlic, minced
- 1 tablespoon ground cumin
- 1 tablespoon ground coriander
- 1 teaspoon ground cinnamon
- 1 teaspoon ground turmeric
- 1/2 teaspoon cayenne pepper (adjust to taste)
- 1 cup chicken broth
- 1/2 cup dried apricots, halved
- 1/2 cup green olives, pitted
- 2 tablespoons honey
- Salt and pepper to taste
- Fresh cilantro or parsley for garnish

For the Couscous:
- 2 cups couscous
- 2 cups chicken broth
- 1 tablespoon olive oil
- Salt to taste

Instructions:

1. Hibiscus-Infused Chicken Tagine:
1. In a large bowl, marinate chicken thighs in hibiscus tea for at least 1 hour.
2. In a tagine or large, heavy-bottomed pot, heat olive oil over medium heat.
3. Sauté chopped onions and minced garlic until softened.
4. Add marinated chicken thighs, cumin, coriander, cinnamon, turmeric, cayenne pepper, salt, and pepper. Brown the chicken on all sides.
5. Pour in chicken broth, add dried apricots, green olives, and honey. Stir to combine.
6. Cover and simmer on low heat for 45-50 minutes or until the chicken is tender and cooked through.
7. Garnish with fresh cilantro or parsley before serving.

2. Couscous:
1. In a separate pot, bring chicken broth and olive oil to a boil.
2. Stir in couscous, cover, and remove from heat. Let it steam for 5 minutes.
3. Fluff the couscous with a fork and add salt to taste.

3. Assembling:
1. Arrange the Hibiscus-Infused Chicken Tagine on a large serving platter.
2. Serve the tagine alongside a generous portion of fluffy couscous.
3. Garnish with additional fresh cilantro or parsley for an elegant touch.

This Moroccan-inspired dish combines the rich, floral notes of hibiscus with aromatic spices, creating a sophisticated and flavorful chicken tagine. Accompanied by perfectly cooked couscous, this dish is well-suited for a formal celebration.

## Hibiscus-Infused Quinoa Salad

Ingredients:

- 1 cup quinoa, rinsed
- 2 cups water
- 1/4 cup dried hibiscus petals
- 1/4 cup chopped fresh cucumber
- 1/4 cup cherry tomatoes, halved
- 2 tablespoons extra virgin olive oil
- 1 tablespoon hibiscus tea (brewed and cooled)
- 1 tablespoon fresh lemon juice
- Salt and pepper to taste
- Fresh mint leaves for garnish (optional)

Instructions:

1. Infusing Quinoa:
   - In a saucepan, bring 2 cups of water to a boil.
   - Add dried hibiscus petals to the boiling water, reduce heat, and let it simmer for 5 minutes.
   - Strain the hibiscus tea, then return it to the saucepan.
   - Add rinsed quinoa to the hibiscus tea, bring back to a boil, then reduce heat, cover, and simmer for 15 minutes or until the quinoa is cooked and water is absorbed.
   - Fluff the quinoa with a fork and let it cool.

2. Assembling the Salad:
   - In a large bowl, combine the cooled hibiscus-infused quinoa, chopped cucumber, and cherry tomatoes.
   - In a small bowl, whisk together extra virgin olive oil, hibiscus tea, fresh lemon juice, salt, and pepper.
   - Drizzle the dressing over the quinoa mixture and toss until well combined.

3. Garnish:
   - Garnish with fresh mint leaves for a burst of freshness and added aroma.
   - Serve chilled or at room temperature as a side dish for the tagine.

## Hibiscus-Infused Khobz with Orange Zest

Our Hibiscus-Infused Khobz with Orange Zest is a masterpiece of Moroccan-inspired bread, designed to elevate your dining experience. This soft and aromatic Khobz carries the delicate notes of hibiscus, offering a subtle floral undertone that intertwines with the citrusy brightness of orange zest. The result is a bread that not only complements the savory richness of a tagine but also stands out as a unique and flavorful side.

**Historical Nuances:**
Khobz, a staple in Moroccan cuisine, has deep historical roots. Traditionally prepared and enjoyed in communal settings, this unleavened flatbread symbolizes the importance of sharing meals. The addition of hibiscus, a flower with a rich history in various culinary traditions globally, pays homage to Morocco's historic connections to trade routes and diverse cultural influences.

**Why Hibiscus?**
The incorporation of hibiscus petals into the Khobz brings more than just a burst of color. Hibiscus has been used historically for its health benefits and unique flavor profile. In this bread, it adds a subtle tanginess and a hint of floral elegance, creating a harmonious marriage with the spices of the tagine. Beyond flavor, hibiscus is known for its vibrant hue, turning the Khobz into a visual delight that complements the vibrant palette of Moroccan cuisine.

**Pairing with Tagine:**
The Hibiscus-Infused Khobz is not just bread; it's a companion to the Hibiscus-Infused Chicken Tagine. As you tear into the soft, warm Khobz, its floral and citrus notes dance alongside the savory and aromatic flavors of the tagine. The hibiscus provides a refreshing contrast, allowing your palate to explore a range of tastes with every bite.

**Perfect Complement:**
This bread is more than a side; it's a perfect complement to the communal spirit of Moroccan dining. As you break bread with loved ones over a steaming tagine, the Hibiscus-Infused Khobz becomes a symbol of shared experiences, connecting the past with the present in a celebration of flavors and togetherness.

### Ingredients:

- 4 cups all-purpose flour
- 1 tablespoon dried hibiscus petals (finely ground)
- 1 tablespoon sugar
- 1 tablespoon orange zest
- 1 tablespoon active dry yeast
- 1 ½ cups warm water
- 2 tablespoons olive oil
- 1 teaspoon salt
- Additional olive oil for brushing

### Instructions:

1. Activate the Yeast:
   - In a small bowl, dissolve sugar in warm water.
   - Sprinkle the active dry yeast over the water, stir gently, and let it sit for 5-10 minutes until frothy.

2. Prepare the Dough:
   - In a large mixing bowl, combine the flour, ground hibiscus petals, orange zest, and salt.
   - Make a well in the center and pour in the activated yeast mixture and olive oil.
   - Mix the ingredients until a dough forms.

3. Knead and Rise:
   - Turn the dough out onto a floured surface and knead for about 8-10 minutes until it becomes smooth and elastic.
   - Place the dough in a lightly oiled bowl, cover it with a damp cloth, and let it rise in a warm place for 1-1.5 hours or until doubled in size.

4. Shape and Second Rise:
   - Preheat the oven to 400°F (200°C).
   - Punch down the risen dough and divide it into small rounds (about the size of a tennis ball).
   - Shape each round into a flat disk and place on a baking sheet.
   - Cover and let the shaped dough rise for an additional 30 minutes.

5. Bake:
   - Brush the tops of the shaped dough with olive oil.
   - Bake in the preheated oven for 15-20 minutes or until the khobz turns golden brown.

6. Cool and Serve:
   - Allow the hibiscus-infused Khobz to cool on a wire rack.
   - Serve the bread warm with the Hibiscus-Infused Chicken Tagine for a delightful dining experience.

Odd Ingredient Note: Feel free to add a tablespoon of finely chopped preserved lemons for a unique twist. Preserved lemons bring a tangy and slightly salty flavor that complements the floral notes of hibiscus and the citrusy aroma of orange zest.

## Quick Hibiscus-Infused Preserved Lemons

By blending organic lemons with a zesty mix of dried hibiscus petals, cinnamon, cloves, and bay leaves, this quick and easy recipe transforms a classic condiment into a flavor-packed sensation. Perfect for adding a tangy, floral essence to tagines, salads, and more, these preserved lemons offer a visually stunning and uniquely nuanced twist to elevate your dishes.

### Ingredients:

- 4-6 organic lemons
- 1/4 cup kosher salt
- 2 tbsp dried hibiscus petals
- 1 cinnamon stick
- 3-4 cloves
- 1-2 bay leaves
- Sterilized glass jar

### Instructions:

1. Prepare Lemons:
   - Wash and quarter lemons, leaving the base intact.

2. Create Spice Mix:
   - Mix salt, hibiscus petals, cinnamon, cloves, and bay leaves.

3. Stuff Lemons:
   - Sprinkle spice mix inside lemons and place in the jar.

4. Layering:
   - Add spice mix between layers and hibiscus petals for visual appeal.

5. Seal and Store:
   - Seal jar and let sit at room temperature for a day.
   - Flip jar and refrigerate for at least three weeks.

6. Usage:
   - Rinse off excess salt before use.
   - Finely chop preserved lemon peel for a unique flavor boost in dishes.

# HIBISCUS: FINAL THOUGHTS

In the world of gastronomy, hibiscus stands as a versatile and vibrant companion, gracing a myriad of realms from drinks to cocktails, home spa rituals, home care, and celebratory occasions. Throughout the ages and across cultures, hibiscus has been revered for its captivating floral notes and multifaceted applications.

In the realm of beverages, the infusion of hibiscus petals transcends mere refreshment, lending a tart and aromatic profile to teas, lemonades, and mocktails alike. Its rich ruby hue, reminiscent of sunsets, adds an aesthetic allure, making every sip a visual and sensory delight. Across continents and epochs, cultures have harnessed hibiscus in their cups, infusing ancient traditions with a touch of modern allure.

Venturing into mixology, hibiscus plays the role of a spirited muse, elevating cocktails to new heights. Its unique flavor profile adds depth and complexity to libations, making it a favored choice for those seeking an exotic twist to their libations. From tropical punches to sophisticated concoctions, hibiscus has found a place in glasses raised in toasts worldwide.

Beyond the realms of gastronomy, hibiscus transcends into the realm of self-care and home spa rituals. With its soothing and nourishing properties, hibiscus petals find their way into facial toners, bath salts, and relaxing pillow mists, offering a holistic approach to beauty and well-being. The ancient echoes of cultures embracing hibiscus for its skincare benefits reverberate through time, connecting past and present in a fragrant tapestry.

In the realm of home care, hibiscus takes on a new role as a natural and aromatic ally. From scented candles to linen sprays, hibiscus transforms living spaces into sanctuaries of tranquility. Its rich history as a symbol of prosperity and good fortune makes it a cherished element in homes, resonating with the belief that the essence of hibiscus brings positivity and joy.

As we celebrate life's milestones, hibiscus unfurls its petals in a myriad of celebratory uses. From adorning culinary creations in festive feasts to gracing gift packages with bath salts and books on its versatile applications, hibiscus becomes a symbol of joy and shared experiences. Its historical presence in ceremonies and celebrations worldwide reflects a universal appreciation for the elegance and vibrancy it imparts.

In conclusion, the enchanting journey with hibiscus traverses not only through culinary landscapes but also into the realms of self-care, home care, and jubilant celebrations. As we explore the myriad ways in which hibiscus has woven itself into the fabric of human experience, we extend our heartfelt gratitude for joining us on this fragrant and flavorful odyssey. Thank you for embracing the beauty and versatility of hibiscus – a timeless companion in our cups, our rituals, and our moments of celebration.

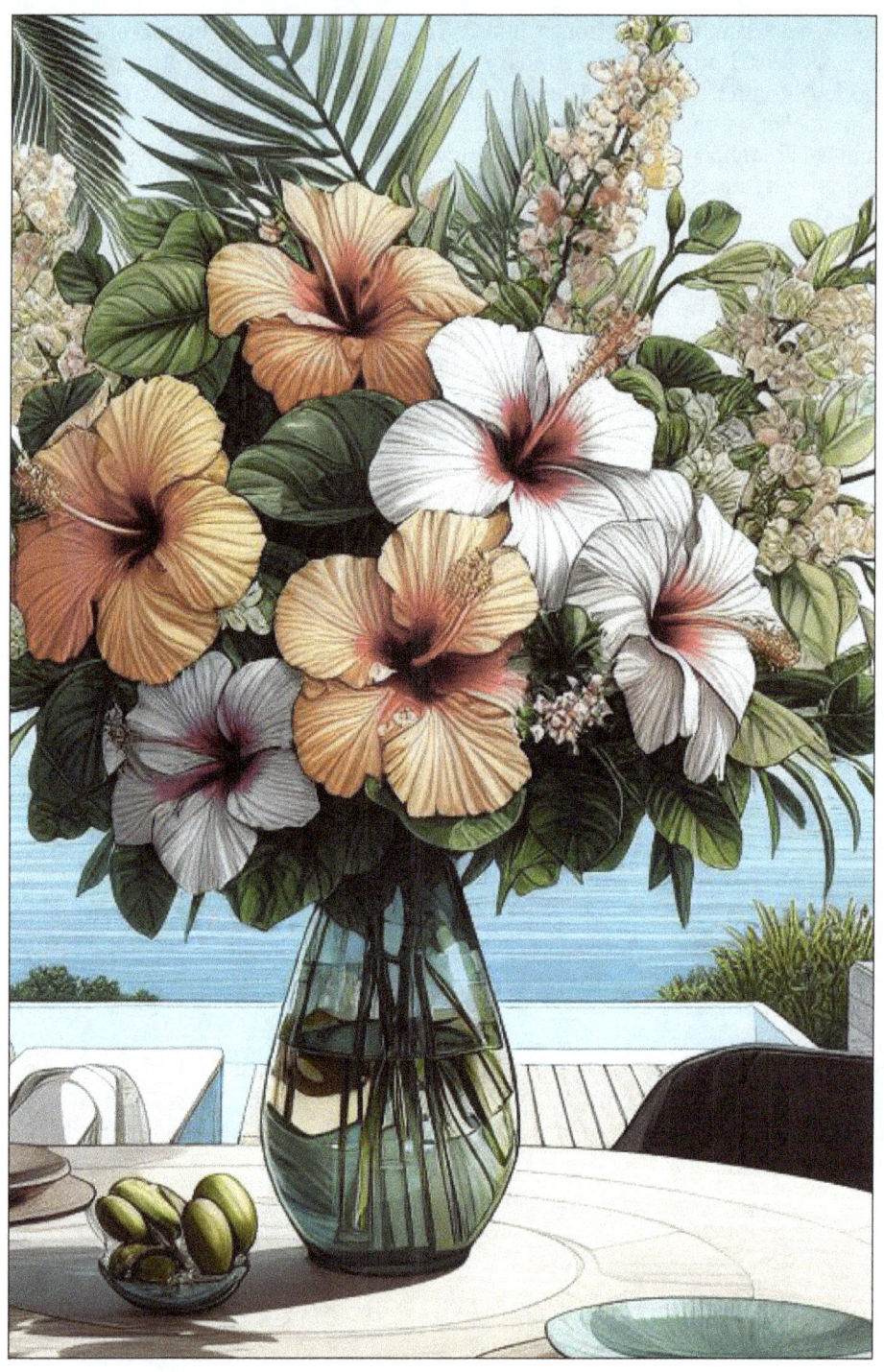

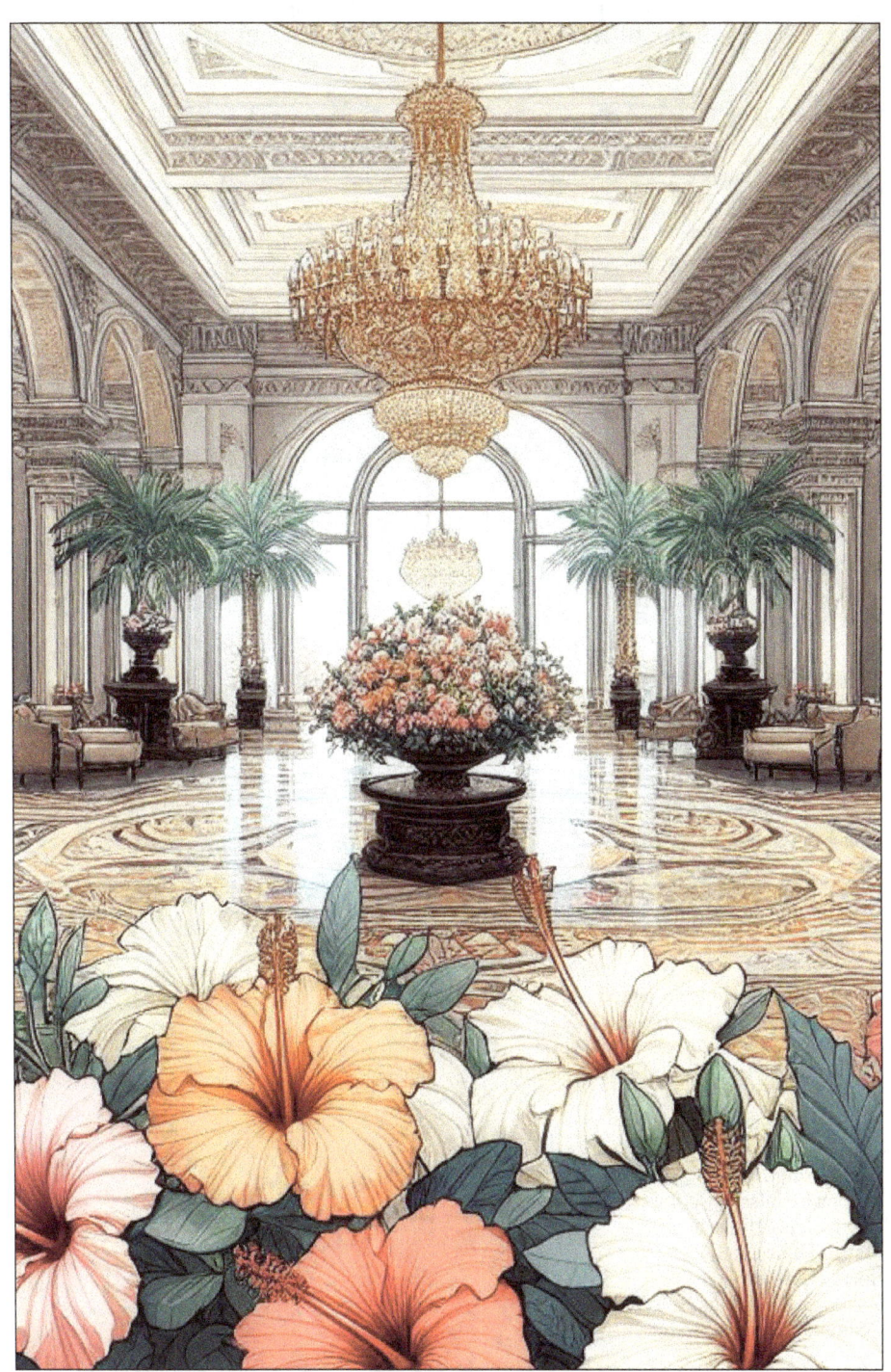

# Index of Recipes, Formulas and Procedures

**Hibiscus Drinks:**

| | |
|---|---|
| Classic Hibiscus Iced Tea | 1 |
| Hibiscus Lemonade | 2 |
| Hibiscus Mint Limeade | 3 |
| Sparkling Hibiscus Water | 4 |
| Hibiscus Ginger Ale | 5 |
| Hibiscus Arnold Palmer | 6 |
| Hibiscus Agua Fresca | 7 |
| Hibiscus Blueberry Sparkler | 8 |
| Coconut Hibiscus Cooler | 9 |
| Hibiscus and Basil Lemon Fizz | 10 |
| Hibiscus Rosemary Spritzer | 11 |
| Spiced Hibiscus Chai | 12 |
| Hibiscus Green Tea Blend | 13 |
| Hibiscus Pineapple Punch | 14 |
| Hibiscus Cranberry Virgin Cocktail | 15 |

**Hibiscus Smoothies:**

| | |
|---|---|
| Tropical Hibiscus Smoothie | 17 |
| Berry Hibiscus Smoothie Bowl | 18 |
| Citrus Hibiscus Bliss Smoothie | 19 |
| Hibiscus Peach Passion Smoothie | 20 |
| Minty Watermelon Hibiscus Smoothie | 21 |
| Creamy Hibiscus Avocado Smoothie | 22 |
| Hibiscus Banana Berry Blast | 23 |
| Mango Tango Hibiscus Smoothie | 24 |
| Hibiscus Pomegranate Power Smoothie | 25 |
| Vanilla Hibiscus Protein Smoothie | 26 |
| Chocolate Hibiscus Delight Smoothie | 27 |
| Hibiscus Spinach Detox Smoothie | 28 |
| Coconut Berry Hibiscus Smoothie | 29 |
| Hibiscus Matcha Fusion Smoothie | 30 |
| Cherry Almond Hibiscus Smoothie | 31 |
| Savory Hibiscus Tomato Basil Smoothie | 32 |

**Hibiscus Mocktails:**

| | |
|---|---|
| Hibiscus Sparkler | 35 |
| Tropical Hibiscus Cooler | 36 |
| Passionfruit Hibiscus Fizz | 37 |
| Mango Hibiscus Splash | 38 |
| Berry Hibiscus Crush | 39 |
| Cucumber Hibiscus Refresher | 40 |
| Coconut Hibiscus Elixir | 41 |

Blueberry Basil Hibiscus Bliss 42
Ginger Lemongrass Hibiscus Infusion 43
Pomegranate Hibiscus Breeze 44

**Hibiscus Cocktails:**

Hibiscus Rose Martini 46
Passion Hibiscus Margarita 47
Coconut Hibiscus Mojito 48
Spicy Hibiscus Pineapple Punch 49
Blue Lagoon Hibiscus Fizz 50
Mango Habanero Hibiscus Splash 51
Cucumber Basil Hibiscus Sling 52
Hibiscus Paloma 53
Smoky Hibiscus Mezcal Mule 54

**Tinctures and Elixirs:**

Hibiscus Heart Health Elixir 60
Digestive Hibiscus Bitters Recipe 61
Enhanced Pacific Island Digestive Tincture 62
Hibiscus Hormonal Balance Tincture Recipe 63
Hibiscus Immune Elixir 64
Hibiscus Joint Relief Elixir 65
Hibiscus Respiratory Tincture 66
Hibiscus Sleep Aid Elixir 67
Hibiscus Lavender Sleep Elixir 68
Hibiscus Digestive Tincture with Traditional Chinese Medicine (TCM) Ingredients 69
Hibiscus Skin Radiance Elixir 70

**Home Spa:**

Hibiscus and Green Tea Face Toner Ice Cubes 74
Hibiscus and Honey Lip Balm 75
Hibiscus and Chamomile Eye Pillow 76
Hibiscus and Peppermint Cooling Face Gel 77
Hibiscus and Matcha Green Tea Face Scrub 78
Hibiscus and Ylang-Ylang Relaxing Pillow Mist 79
Hibiscus and Oatmeal Face Mask 80
Hibiscus and Lemon Cuticle Oil 81
Hibiscus Facial Steam 82
Hibiscus and Green Clay Face Pack 83
Hibiscus and Rose Petal Bath Salts 84
Hibiscus and Honey Face Wash 85
Hibiscus and Aloe Vera Cooling Gel 86
Hibiscus and Red Wine Anti-Aging Serum 87
Hibiscus and Turmeric Brightening Face Elixir 88
Hibiscus and Kakadu Plum Dark Spot Corrector 89

| | |
|---|---|
| Volcanic Ash and Hibiscus Facial Mask | 90 |
| Hibiscus Bath Soak | 92 |
| Hibiscus-Lemon Foot Soak | 94 |
| Hibiscus Citrus Bliss Bath Crystals | 95 |
| Hibiscus Scented Candles | 97 |
| Hibiscus and Jasmine Scented Milk Bath | 98 |
| Hibiscus Citrus Oatmeal Soap Bar | 99 |
| Hibiscus Bath Bomb | 99 |

**Household Hibiscus:**

| | |
|---|---|
| Hibiscus All-Purpose Cleaner | 101 |
| Hibiscus Linen Spray | 102 |
| Hibiscus Dish Soap | 103 |
| Hibiscus Carpet Freshener | 104 |
| Hibiscus Furniture Polish | 105 |
| Hibiscus Stain Remover | 106 |
| Hibiscus Pot and Pan Scrub | 107 |
| Hibiscus Deodorizing Bags | 108 |

**Gifts + Celebrations:**

| | |
|---|---|
| Hibiscus-Scented Cologne | 111 |
| Hibiscus Shaving Cream | 112 |
| Hibiscus Perfume | 113 |
| Hibiscus-Infused Chocolate Truffles | 114 |
| Grilled Hibiscus-Glazed Chicken Skewers with Pineapple Mango Salsa | 115 |
| Moroccan-Inspired Hibiscus-Infused Chicken Tagine | 116 |
| Hibiscus-Infused Quinoa Salad | 117 |
| Hibiscus-Infused Khobz with Orange Zest | 118 |
| Quick Hibiscus-Infused Preserved Lemons | 119 |

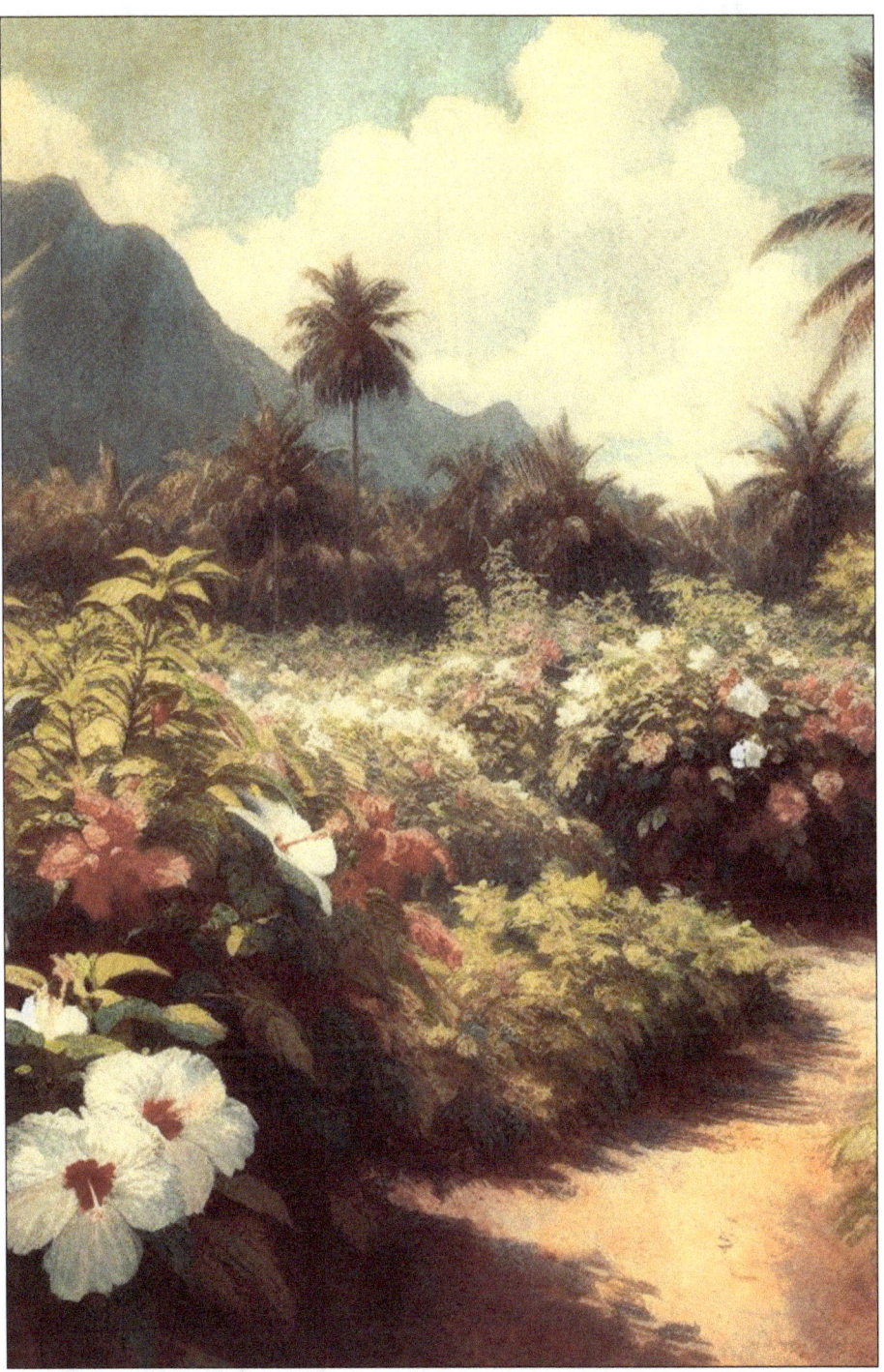